180° Privacy

Disclaimer,

180° is committed to protecting your privacy. We collect personal information solely to provide
our services and products to you. We do not share, sell, or rent your personal information with third parties, except in the following circumstances:

To comply with legal requirements or to respond to a subpoena or other legal process.

To protect the rights, property, or safety of 180°, our customers, or others.

To provide your information to trusted partners who work on our behalf, under confidentiality agreements. We implement reasonable security measures to protect your personal information from unauthorized access, use, or disclosure.

The content of this program, including text, images, and other materials are the property of 180° or its licensors. You may not reproduce, modify, display, sell, or distribute the content, or use it for any public or commercial purpose, without our prior written permission.

The 180° Name, logo, and intellectual property is the exclusive property of Arm Leg Leg Arm Head.Trademark 180° All other trademarks, service marks, and trade names are the property of their respective owners of Arm Leg.

By using our services and products, you agree to our privacy disclaimer and copyright notice. If you do not agree, please do not use our services and products.

Note: This is a sample and should be reviewed and customized according to specific needs and legal requirements.

Privacy Disclaimer

180° is committed to protecting your privacy. We collect personal information solely to provide our services and products to you. We do not share, sell, or rent your personal information with third parties, except in the following circumstances:

© 2024 180° All Rights Reserved Courtesy Of ARM LEG LEG ARM HEAD.TM
THIS BOOK WAS RESEARCHED BY MIKE MONTERO COURTESY OF ARM LEG LEG ARM HEAD.TM

180°

is a 90 pounds 90-day weight loss wellness guide as a perfect guide to unlocking the power within with exercise and diet to obtain a

healthy lifestyle and your Ideal Physique" As well as the Mental psyche for an elevated mindset to becoming the best version of you. According to information, I've gathered over years of experience and research. I believe 180° will educate readers and anyone who is seeking a life-changing experience with a basic diet and workout plan to start and mindset tools to obtain the desired weight loss of 90 pounds in 90 days. When you apply these tools to your everyday life you feel better and think better. When you apply this 90 pounds in 90 days program you are doing a 180-degree turnaround in your life and daily habits and or routine. Smile things are about to turn around if you're serious and dedicated to the new journey and stay consistent.

This is a guide for Highly Motivated People seeking to better their lives and become the best you. Broken down to a perfect science.

Explanation Dialog:

Are you ready to achieve your dream body with a 90-pound weight loss plan in 90 days? Completing your 180° turn? Then spreading the word of this progress, then seeing your process come back for a complete 360-

degree circle of positivity. Gaining self-awareness, and using each one teaches one mindset that will create a Mandela effect changing the future with the best positive outcome possible. This comprehensive program is designed to help you lose weight, build lean muscle, and boost your overall health and mindset. Thank GOD,
We have finally arrived.
Here's what you'll get: "Hey there,
My name is MIKE MONTERO from Santa of Clarita Valley, CA, and welcome to 180° The circle beside the zero represents degrees so 180 degrees you're about to do the opposite of your daily routine! 90-pound weight loss in just 90 days. Now let's start with a little backstory before we get into the meat of this manuscript.

Growing up wasn't a cakewalk. I didn't have an easy life but along my journey.
I learned consistency and hard work, along with my reaction to good or bad situations, determined the outcome of whatever the results were. When facing life's obstacles,
I learned the more I kept a positive attitude without expectations. Meaning looking at the brighter side of things.
I noticed there was always a better outcome,
then when I reacted negatively, taking a closer look at my part,

not holding on to resentment, not judging anyone else, and being a rock for those in my family and friend groups.

Taking the time to say nice things to people while being patient with others. Letting someone go first at the stop sign. Addressing issues unbiasedly. My timing became perfect and I was able to see the blessing and gifts GOD, the Universe, Spirit or my higher power had in store for me.

All the places I've been and programs I've been a part of, for training purposes, reward or punishment. I have always taken advantage of all outlets that were offered to me to make me a better person and or to build my skills. I've also always made the best of every situation and worked hard to better myself by using obstacles as lessons when I faced any problems, usually that were of my own doing whether good or bad turning a negative into a positive.

I've always taken advantage of the outlets that were offered to me. Jumping into every opportunity that educated me and trained me to be successful and a better high-performance individual.

This is the first look into my definition of knowledge, wisdom, and understanding that brought me freedom, power and refinement, equality, becoming GOD's conscience while building The new me and destroying old thoughts and habits while training myself to lose 90 pounds in 90 days a new man was born.

The results were more than I could have wished for, I truly am grateful to GOD for this experience.

Now what has taken me a lifetime to understand. I have taken the time to break down this process for you, practically and easily for you to process, so you may change your diet and mindset. The new habits I present to you are gathered through research,
facts and statistics of the body and mindset that produce results if you work this regimen and stay consistent.

Everything in 180° is through my study as well as my own life experiences, questions I've had and had to answer with research and applying them in my own life, has shifted my own thought patterns, perception, routines, and eating habits, with a diet plan that has lead to a successful lifestyle and a goal-accomplishing attitude.

More or less these are just important things a human being can do that will help your health physically as well as mindset raising your vibration while setting milestones on a journey of self-improvement and spiritual growth. Mainly by being open to change, and training your sub-conscience to get into a better routine and great eating habits.
Fasting, and detoxifying your body is a start to re-setting your intake of food in your normal day-to-day life that can cause long-term health problems. So when you fast you're cleansing your body of all the old toxins that you are so used to in your day-to-day lives.

When you think about it, your body is like an engine. What does it take for an engine to run great?

Easy Answer, it needs oil, coolant, and gas to run. Every so many miles you have to flush the system and add new fluids.

That is the same for our bodies in a sense, when you think about it.

The Best way to change our fluids is to stay hydrated. Our bodies are a large percentage of water, so look into foods that are healthy for your daily meals and change your eating habits, meaning how much food you consume.

A healthy diet is 75 percent of the journey to a healthy body and workout plan.

Now some people prefer to be muscular. Putting weight on with muscle mass has long-term effects; it can damage your joints, with the continued strain of the weight you add to your body in such a fast time. So before you try and bulk up, Please see your doctor so

He/She may give you the proper supplements to build up your joint strength before lifting to add muscle mass. This book is not for bulking up, this is a diet weight loss workout plan for a height-to-weight ratio.

As well as a mindset-building guide for those seeking a better mind and body through working out and eating the right foods.

When you inner-stand a few simple steps. Then you add on to what I am showing you,
With your research, and planning. You will be amazed at your willingness, strength, and power, as well as
YOUR RESULTS!
	You will Thank GOD every day,
that you have done a complete 180° into the healthy lifestyle you so desired before you started.
You will gain self-knowledge of health workouts that affect each muscle group, and with your research, into foods and exercises,
you will be focused on your self-improvement.
Which will keep your idle minds busy, and give you confidence in yourself, inside and out.
 It takes heart to change your life, it takes dedication to switch your normal routine and last but not least it takes consistency to keep on trudging along when we can't see the quick results to the finish line.
Looking for new ways to exercise learning about what food to eat and how to cook then and prepare your meals will help you stay excited for self-improvement.
If you're looking to have ripped washboard abs, you must eat a lean diet, less fatty foods, and watch and count calories. I fluctuated my weight over the years and the weight, and I felt at my best and youthful with the least amount of resistance in movement and breathing,
When I used the height-to-weight ratio, a list of height-to-

weight ratios for men and women is also in this book in later pages. Everyone has their preference. You may add on to your preferences. This is just a blueprint I've created for those people out there who want to change their mindset, and physical appearance or lose 90 pounds in 90 days for a 180° life-changing turn around.

For the next 90 days. I want you to listen and only watch positive inspirational videos or clips, movies, and music content. What we are doing is changing our mindset. Now I believe our minds are like antennas, what we hear, and see is what we perceive and speak. By using this method we are rewiring our sub-conscience to think and react in a positive manner letting go of our old ways of thinking. Train your mind to stay on the brighter side of every situation, we then begin to change our perception thus creating a shift in our reality in real-time. For example, just because you woke up late doesn't mean you have to rush or feel bad about it,
Sometimes we mess up our plans by going to bed late, oversleeping, overworking ourselves, etc. Then we rush in haste, now everything else becomes off in our daily routine. *Am I Right?!*

Things just seem all shaken up from that point, we feel like our whole day is upside down like a tornado threw off our whole day. I suggest just accepting it. A missed opportunity is not always a bad thing. When it comes to working at a job you already have or a class you are in, I suggest you just reset, forgive yourself, and take the time to do your daily preparations that make you feel your best. DO what usually helps you perform at your best.

We make the mental decision or choice to be happy or react to situations life throws at us positively or negatively.

So just take a pause and think about what you're about to say before you say it,
and have a good day. Eventually, your brain will catch on and become more aware and awake to catching your character defects. When you do what is normal to you like when you overreact to situations or replying to something that doesn't serve your higher purpose, like impulsive mannerisms. In my opinion, that's walking in God's will. No one is perfect, it's our imperfections that make us beautiful sometimes, so be easy on yourself. Do your best to correct any negativity. Try to set boundaries and never settle for less than your worth.

Honestly, you won't believe how many of us are not really paying attention to what others are doing. Most of us are caught up in our own daily lives, even noticing our surroundings. After a bit of practice, you will become awake to everything in your circumference. Thus the saying, I'm awake. If you're late you wouldn't believe what a simple call can do. Making courtesy calls and being kind can help your immediate relationships with friends, a boss, your coworkers, or whomever you choose to be meeting, working for, or any opportunity that you have scheduled at that moment in time.

When you think about it, every show must go on and just like the water in the ocean the tides will adjust themselves immediately. Most of the time we overthink about the past which creates depression, or our future trip and that causes anxiety. When you create a schedule use the 5 P method *"Proper Planning.*

Prevents Poor Performance."
Look at the world as a test of character. "How will *YOU deal* with obstacles.?"
Will you let things ruin your day or will you let hick-ups in your daily routine roll off your shoulders and be grateful for whatever the world throws at you? For example when you're On your way somewhere and you catch a traffic jam,

Just by being calm and in a peaceful mindset is how you get out of depression, learn to notice your mood change and make up your mind to become instantly happy just start thinking positively. Think of someone who made you laugh or a time when you were happy about something and re-emulate that feeling or that emotion. By doing that you're taking yourself out of your normal subconscious reactions, please understand the subconscious is a lazy part of your mind that just wants to do the easiest things that it's used to. That's how you change your mindset and being in this mindset you will eventually shift your

Negative Thinking into a logical patient positive energy. Thus the saying." Shifting the energy from negative to positive consciousness.

There's a story about the best Archer in all the land, who's doing all these tricks he's at a Renaissance fair showing his talent hitting bulls with every shot and splitting arrows. He's a perfect marksman with a bow and arrow. Well, at the exhibition every time he shot an old man in the background, kept yelling that anybody could do that. It just takes practice. So after the exhibition, the archer went up to the old man and said hey I heard you heckling saying that anybody can do what I can do. I'm the best Archer in the whole world. But the old man simply smiled and said, "I wasn't heckling you, I was just merely stating that anybody who practices like you do, can achieve your skills."   The old man was pouring oils into small bottles and said to the Archer, "Can you pour these jugs into the small bottle?" The Archer tried to give the challenge a try, but he spilled all over the place and got oil everywhere. The old man laughed while taking the jug from the archer. He began to pour into a small bottle without spilling a drop.
He then said to the archer. "You can do this too if you practice like I have."
The moral of the story is anything you do takes time and effort and practice, dedication, consistency, even becoming healthy, fit, a great, person, a great parent, a

great student, or requiring a skill set in any career, you choose as a life passion, with enough practice, you become a master at it.

What am I Getting In Such A Small Book? You ask...

· A personalized workout plan tailored to your height, weight, and fitness goals

· A daily exercise routine that includes a mix of cardio, strength training, and flexibility exercises

· A meal plan that includes healthy, delicious recipes and portion control guidance

· Progress tracking and support from our community of like--

minded individuals

By following Transform 180° you can expect to:

- *Lose 1-2 pounds per week*

- *Gain 1-2 pounds of lean muscle per week*

- Increase your energy levels and overall well-being. ***Don't wait any longer to achieve your ideal physique.***

- Join 180° today and start your 90-day weight loss in 90 days for a 180° journey to a healthier, happier you!"

  Now Let's Start With A Easy Workout Plan:

  Day 1-90: Cardio (10-15) minutes a day. Upper Body

Strength

 Core Strength Training + Lower Body Strength (5 times a week)

 Cardio

 (10-15)minutes, 5 times a week) + Upper Body + Core

 (45-60) minutes in the gym or at home

 Daily pre-workout routine is non negotiable.

 light stretch

 (5- 10) minute jog/treadmill or outside

 This will warm up your muscles before lifting weights please note to try and increase,

 your speed your pace weekly-

 Let's Get Started With Day 1

 Always Start with A

 light stretch before

 (5- 10) minute jog/treadmill or outdoors to warm up increase your speed weekly

Muscle Focus- Back/Chest

start with some wide pull-ups 3 sets to your full max of reps even if you can do it 1 it's ok just do what you can and be patient with yourself

CHEST AND BACK

 (4-5) sets (5-15) reps 30-60 second rest

I do a set of ups or pull-ups in between sets as a rest.

Bench press and seated cable rows are a good starting point for your first week.

I suggest mixing up the chest and back workouts, but it's to everybody's preference, make sure you switch your routine weekly to your lineup of muscle groups.

So if you started Monday on your back and chest the next week, you want to start on a different muscle group on Monday.

I could give you a list of exercises but that would defeat the purpose of your journey.

" Motivated individuals do the work and it feels better once you achieve your success."Mike Montero

So please look up a list of workouts for each muscle group to add to your routines.

Push Pull

Make sure you chose a weight you can do back-to-back reps and sets

We are shocking the muscles and strength-building

Not hanging out and wasting time.

We are busy and focused on the task at hand even if you can just pull off 1 rep just go do a pull-up or push-up.In between or rest no longer than (30-60) seconds.

End every workout with a burnout set of burpees.

Burpees are a full-body workout and incorporate all muscle groups. It's a squat, hands-down in a push-up position. Kick out your feet then do a push-up jump your feet inwards towards your hands and stand up. That's one and you can choose how many push-ups you do.

Day 2 Shoulders/Traps (3-4) sets

 (5-15)reps (30-60) rest in between reps

 Or use that time to do some push-ups or pull-ups face pull /Trap bar shrugs to start with

Day3 biceps/triceps (3-4) reps (5-15) reps

 (30 -60) sec rest in between reps or push up pull-ups

 Curls/overhead triceps extensions

"Learning the different Exercises is key.

So you can switch up the days of your routine and exercises so your body doesn't get used to the same thing that's how you shock the muscles "

 Mike Montero

Day4 most important day Legs are your foundation. The core is the center of your strength.

 Legs/ core

(3-4)sets (5-15) reps

(30-60) sec rest

 Leg presses

 You can also do your calves on the leg press before each rep Military 3 count crunches Right, Left,Middle

Day5 Cardio and bodyweight exercise Jog or run in place.

 high knees up

 Crawl push ups

Pull-ups Dips

 (2-4)sets

(5-15)reps
 (30-60) rest in between reps
keep in mind to breath and keep your heart rate up for max fat burning later in the read you will learn the importance of breathing and the way your body burns fat and reforms it self to your new body
so make sure you read this whole book before you start your routine and new habits of health and diet.
Day6 rest -
 Day7 rest-

I usually would play basketball on Saturdays or just spend the day stretching. I would work myself so hard my muscles would go into convulsions at night so I would have to stretch a lot, but I never wanted to be bulky or have a massive weight. I worked out to be athletic agile and fit
exercise is important but the most important is your diet. Let me repeat the most important part of getting fit is your diet plan. A healthy diet plan is the most important part of your results.
So let me reiterate. When shocking your muscles make sure you switch your muscle groups days and weekly to shock and confuse the muscles for maximum strength building. Your muscles have memory, so let's say you were a fit person before you gained weight or fell off the workout wagon, at one time you had a six pack and you

had nice arms. Once you start working out again, a week into 180° you will notice the difference because your muscle has memory.
Breathing practice -

 Sometimes we work out and breathe wrong so you want to practice
your breathing skills sometimes we even forget to breathe and we don't even notice it or during exercises, we hold our breath.
 Take the time to practice your breathing and get in the habits of breathing correctly when you breathe in, it should look like your stomach is filled up or pushed out and when you breathe out, your stomach should be sucked in, like you're touching your ribs with your stomach yoga is a great place to learn how to stretch and breath release stress and tension.
I *go to my favorite yoga place. I just love the people and vibration in the rooms here.*
 Thermal Horizon Wellness Center
25830 McBean Pkwy Valencia, CA 91355
 "Just tell them Mike Montero sent you!"
It's located in the greater Los Angeles area
in My AWESOME home town of Santa Clarita Ca
(5 times a week) focus 15-20 minutes of meditation and practice your breathing in thru the nose slowly out thru the nose. That's called breath control calming and controlling

your heart rate. after each set deep breath in thru the nose out thru the mouth... aaaaaahhhhh releasing all negative energy.. Namaste
Meal Plan:

Your diet plan is the most important part of your routine, Possessing the ability to change your old eating habits takes discipline Start off eating half of what your normal portions are
 Light breakfast light lunch and a good portion dinner before 6 pm give your body time to digest your food sleep on your back
This will help clear your sinus cavity. Also when you sleep on your side, you get knots in your shoulders, especially when you're working out because you're restricting the blood flow to your muscles and that creates knots in your muscles.
Alright, let's start with Day 1 of our 90-day meal plan. Here's a sample menu for the day:
Day 1:
 Breakfast:
 - Scrambled eggs (2 eggs) with spinach and whole-grain toast Lunch:
 - Grilled chicken breast (4 oz) with quinoa and roasted vegetables Dinner:
 - Baked salmon (6 oz) with sweet potato and steamed broccoli

How does this plan look for Day 1? We can continue this for the next 89 days with more tasty and healthy options!

Let's keep the healthy meal train rolling with Day 2 of our plan!
Here's a delicious and nutritious menu for you:
Day 2:
 Breakfast:
 - Greek yogurt with mixed berries and a sprinkle of granola Lunch:
 - Turkey and avocado wrap with a side salad
 Dinner:
 - Stir-fried tofu with mixed vegetables and brown rice
How does this Day 2 plan sound? We're on a roll with these healthy meals!
Alright! Let's dive into Day 3 of our meal plan. Here are some tasty and healthy options for your meals:
Day 3:
 Breakfast:
 - Oatmeal with sliced bananas and a drizzle of honey
 Lunch:
 - Grilled shrimp salad with mixed greens and a balsamic vinaigrette Dinner:
 - Lean beef stir-fry with bell peppers and brown rice
How does this plan for Day 3 look? Keep up the good work with these nutritious choices!

Let's keep the healthy meal plan going with Day 4! Here's a delicious menu for you:
Day 4:
 Breakfast:
 - Smoothie with spinach, banana, and almond milk
 Lunch:
 - Quinoa salad with chickpeas, cucumber, and feta cheese Dinner:

- Grilled salmon with asparagus and wild rice
How does this plan for Day 4 sound to you? We're on a roll with these nutritious meals!
Let's keep the healthy meal streak going with Day 5! Here's a tasty menu for you:
Day 5:
 Breakfast:
 - Avocado toast with a poached egg on top
 Lunch:
 - Lentil soup with a side of whole-grain bread
 Dinner:
 - Grilled chicken skewers with zucchini and couscous

How does this Day 5 plan sound to you? These meals are not only delicious but also packed with nutrients!

Alright! Let's continue with Day 6 of our meal plan. Here are some tasty and healthy options for your meals:

Day 6:

Breakfast:

- Chia seed pudding with mixed berries

Lunch:

- Turkey and avocado wrap with a side salad

Dinner:

- Baked cod with roasted Brussels sprouts and quinoa

How does this plan for Day 6 look to you? Keep up the great work with these nutritious choices!

Alright, Let's wrap up the week with Day 7 of our meal plan. Here's a delicious and healthy menu for you:

Day 7: Breakfast:

- Whole grain toast with smashed avocado and a sprinkle of red pepper flakes
 Lunch:
 - Grilled chicken salad with mixed greens, cherry tomatoes, and a light vinaigrette
Dinner:
 - Veggie stir-fry with tofu and quinoa
How does this plan for Day 7 sound to you? You've been doing great with these nutritious meals!
Here are some more little ideas

- · Breakfast: Overnight oats with fruit and nuts

- · Lunch: Grilled chicken salad with avocado and whole grain crackers

- · Dinner: Baked salmon with quinoa and steamed vegetables

- · Snacks: Greek yogurt with berries, carrot sticks with hummus

 Remember, consistency and patience are key. Stick to the program, and you'll be on your way to a transformed body in just 90 days!"

 clarifying that the meal portions I provided earlier are per serving. Here's a revised breakdown of the daily

meal plan with serving sizes:
Breakfast

- · 2 whole eggs (140 calories, 12g protein)

- · 1 cup cooked oatmeal (150 calories, 3g protein)

- · 1 banana (100 calories, 2g protein)
Total Calories: 390 Total Protein: 17g

Serving Size: 1 meal Lunch

- · 4 oz grilled chicken breast (120 calories, 25g protein)

- · 1 cup mixed greens salad (20 calories, 2g protein)

- · 1/2 cup cooked quinoa (100 calories, 4g protein)

- · 1 avocado (140 calories, 3g protein)
Total Calories: 380 Total Protein: 34g

Serving Size: 1 meal Dinner

- · 6 oz grilled salmon (210 calories, 35g protein)

- · 1 cup cooked brown rice (110 calories, 2g protein)

- · 1 cup steamed broccoli (55 calories, 2g protein)

Total Calories: 375 Total Protein: 39g

Serving Size: 1 meal Snacks

- · 1 small apple (95 calories, 0g protein)

- · 1 oz almonds (160 calories, 6g protein)

Total Calories: 255 Total Protein: 6g

Serving Size: 1 snack

Please note that these serving sizes are approximate and may vary based on individual needs. Also, the protein amounts are

approximate and may vary based on specific ingredients and brands used.

Remember to stay hydrated by drinking plenty of water throughout the day. Also, listen to your body and rest when needed. Adjust the workout plan as needed to avoid injury. Consult with a healthcare professional before starting any new diet or exercise program.

Here is an example of a daily log for the 90-day body transformation program:

Day 1-30

· Meal Log

 - Breakfast: Overnight oats with fruit and nuts

 - Lunch: Grilled chicken salad with avocado and whole grain

crackers

 - Dinner: Baked salmon with quinoa and steamed vegetables

 - Snacks: Greek yogurt with berries, carrot sticks with hummus

·

Workout Log

 - Cardio (30 minutes): Treadmill or jogging - Upper Body Strength Training:

- Push-ups (3 sets of 12 reps)

 - Bicep curls (3 sets of 12 reps) - Tricep dips (3 sets of 12 reps)

Day 31-60

· Meal Log

 - Breakfast: Scrambled eggs with whole grain toast and avocado - Lunch: Turkey and avocado wrap with mixed greens

- Dinner: Grilled chicken breast with sweet potato and green
beans
- Snacks: Apple slices with almond butter, protein smoothie
· Workout Log
- Cardio (30 minutes): Cycling or swimming - Lower Body Strength Training:
- Squats (3 sets of 12 reps)
- Lunges (3 sets of 12 reps)
- Calf raises (3 sets of 12 reps)
Day 61-90
·

·

Meal Log
- Breakfast: Greek yogurt with berries and granola
- Lunch: Grilled chicken salad with quinoa and mixed vegetables - Dinner: Baked salmon with brown rice and steamed broccoli
- Snacks: Hard-boiled egg, hummus with carrot and celery sticks
Workout Log
- Cardio (30 minutes): High-intensity interval training (HIIT) - Core Strength Training:
- Plank (3 sets of 30-second hold) - Russian twists (3 sets of 12 reps) - Leg raises (3 sets of 12 reps)

Do not eat the same meal every week this is just to get you on the path on a search for healthy substitutes it will get you involved in your process by learning and researching and finding what you like to what your favorite exercises are depending on your level of knowledge and skill in wellness and fitness keep in mind what you're putting into your body if your losing weight eat half your normal portions of food when losing weight if you choose to eat the food that gave you extra weight you so desire to lose

supplement more food into your diet

 This 180 degree plan is designed for a height to weight ratio the perfect weight to your height

Body Part Focus

. . .

Day 1-90: Upper body (chest, shoulders, triceps) Lower body (legs, glutes, calves)

Core (abs, obliques, lower back) traps triceps, forearms all muscles

Women:

Here are the height-to-weight charts for women and men between 5'0" and 7'0":

Women:

· 5'0" (60 in) - moderate weight: 95-120 lbs; overweight: 125-150 lbs

- · 5'1" (61 in) - moderate weight: 98-123 lbs; overweight: 128-153 lbs

- · 5'2" (62 in) - moderate weight: 101-126 lbs; overweight: 131-156 lbs

· 5'3" (63 in) - moderate weight: 104-129 lbs; overweight: 134-159 lbs

· 5'4" (64 in) - moderate weight: 107-132 lbs; overweight: 137-162 lbs

· 5'5" (65 in) - moderate weight: 110-135 lbs; overweight: 140-165 lbs

· 5'6" (66 in) - moderate weight: 113-138 lbs; overweight: 143-168 lbs

· 5'7" (67 in) - moderate weight: 116-141 lbs; overweight: 146-171 lbs

· 5'8" (68 in) - moderate weight: 119-144 lbs; overweight: 149-174 lbs

· 5'9" (69 in) - moderate weight: 122-147 lbs; overweight: 152-177 lbs

· 5'10" (70 in) - moderate weight: 125-150 lbs; overweight: 155-180 lbs

· 5'11" (71 in) - moderate weight: 128-153 lbs; overweight: 158-183 lbs

· 6'0" (72 in) - moderate weight: 131-156 lbs; overweight: 161-186 lbs

· 6'1" (73 in) - moderate weight: 134-159 lbs; overweight: 164-189 lbs

· 6'2" (74 in) - moderate weight: 137-162 lbs; overweight: 167-192 lbs

· 6'3" (75 in) - moderate weight: 140-165 lbs; overweight: 170-195 lbs

· 6'4" (76 in) - moderate weight: 143-168 lbs; overweight: 173-198 lbs

· 6'5" (77 in) - moderate weight: 146-171 lbs; overweight: 176-201 lbs

· 6'6" (78 in) - moderate weight: 149-174 lbs; overweight: 179-204 lbs

· 6'7" (79 in) - moderate weight: 152-177 lbs; overweight: 182-207 lbs

· 6'8" (80 in) - moderate weight: 155-180 lbs; overweight: 185-210 lbs

· 6'9" (81 in) - moderate weight: 158-183 lbs; overweight: 188-213 lbs

· 6'10" (82 in) - moderate weight: 161-186 lbs; overweight: 191-216 lbs

· 6'11" (83 in) - moderate weight: 164-189 lbs; overweight: 194-219 lbs

· 7'0" (84 in) - moderate weight: 167-192 lbs; overweight: 197-222 lbs

Men:

· 5'0" (60 in) - moderate weight: 104-131 lbs; overweight: 136-157 lbs

· 5'1" (61 in) - moderate weight: 107-134 lbs; overweight: 139-160 lbs

· 5'2" (62 in) - moderate weight: 110-137 lbs; overweight: 142-163 lbs

· 5'3" (63 in) - moderate weight: 113-140 lbs; overweight: 145-166 lbs

· 5'4" (64 in) - moderate weight: 116-143 lbs; overweight: 148-169 lbs

· 5'5" (65 in) - moderate weight: 119-146 lbs; overweight: 151-172 lbs

· 5'6" (66 in) - moderate weight: 122-149 lbs; overweight: 154-175 lbs

· 5'7" (67 in) - moderate weight: 125-152 lbs; overweight: 157-178 lbs

· 5'8" (68 in) - moderate weight: 128-155 lbs; overweight: 160-181 lbs

· 5'9" (69 in) - moderate weight: 131-158 lbs; overweight: 163-184 lbs:

5'10" (70 inches) tall

- · Moderate weight: 134-161 lbs

- · Overweight: 166-186 lbs

- · 5'11" (71 in) - moderate weight: 137-164 lbs; overweight: 169-190 lbs

· 6'0" (72 in) - moderate weight: 140-167 lbs; overweight: 172-195 lbs

· 6'1" (73 in) - moderate weight: 143-170 lbs; overweight: 175-200 lbs

· 6'2" (74 in) - moderate weight: 146-173 lbs; overweight: 178-205 lbs

· 6'3" (75 in) - moderate weight: 149-176 lbs; overweight: 181-210 lbs

· 6'4" (76 in) - moderate weight: 152-179 lbs; overweight: 184-215 lbs

· 6'5" (77 in) - moderate weight: 155-182 lbs; overweight: 187-220 lbs

· 6'6" (78 in) - moderate weight: 158-185 lbs; overweight: 190-225 lbs

· 6'7" (79 in) - moderate weight: 161-188 lbs; overweight: 193-230 lbs

· 6'8" (80 in) - moderate weight: 164-191 lbs; overweight: 196-235 lbs

· 6'9" (81 in) - moderate weight: 167-194 lbs; overweight: 199-240 lbs

· 6'10" (82 in) - moderate weight: 170-197 lbs; overweight: 202-245 lbs

· 6'11" (83 in) - moderate weight: 173-200 lbs; overweight: 205-250 lbs

· 7'0" (84 in) - moderate weight: 176-203 lbs; overweight: 208-255 lbs

Please keep in mind that these are general guidelines and that a healthy weight can vary depending on individual factors such as
muscle mass, bone density, and body composition.
Please note that these are general guidelines and that ideal weight can vary depending on age, muscle mass, bone density, and other factors. It's always best to consult a healthcare professional to determine a healthy weight range.
If you have no weights, there are still many effective ways to work out and achieve a 90-day transformation. Here are some alternate exercises and options:
1. Bodyweight exercises: Squats, push-ups, lunges, planks, tricep dips (using a chair or bench), burpees, etc.
 2. Resistance bands: Portable and lightweight, these provide resistance in various strengths.
3. High-Intensity Interval Training (HIIT): Short bursts of intense exercise (e.g., sprints, jumping jacks, etc.) followed by brief rest periods.
 4. Isometric exercises: Planks, wall sits, glute bridges, etc., which contract muscles without movement.
5. Yoga or Pilates: Modify exercises to suit your fitness level, focusing on strength, flexibility, and core stability.
 6. Cardio exercises: Running, cycling, swimming, dancing, or brisk walking.
7. Home workout programs: Follow along with videos or apps like Nike Training Club, JEFIT, or 7 Minute Workout.

8. Stair climbing: Find a staircase and climb for a great cardio workout.

9. Jump rope: A classic cardio exercise that's easy to do anywhere.

10. Progressive overload: Increase reps, sets, or-duration as you get stronger.

Remember to always listen to your body and start slowly, increasing intensity and difficulty as you progress. Consult a healthcare professional or fitness expert to create a personalized workout plan tailored to your needs and goals.

For busy moms and dads, finding time to exercise can be challenging. Here are some quick and effective workout ideas that can be done in just a few minutes:

1. 7-minute workout: A quick circuit of bodyweight exercises like burpees, jump squats, and mountain climbers.

2. HIIT (High-Intensity Interval Training): Short bursts of intense exercise followed by brief rest periods.

3. Bodyweight exercises: Squats, push-up, lunges, planks, for tricep dips using a chair or bench.

4. Jump rope: A quick cardio workout that can be done in just a few minutes.

5. Stair climbing: Find a staircase and climb for a great cardio workout.

6. Quick yoga flow: A fast-paced yoga routine focusing on strength, flexibility, and breathing.

7. Tabata workout: 20 seconds of all-out effort followed by 10 seconds of rest.

8. Plank jacks: Hold a plank position and jump your feet between different positions.

9. Wall sit: Stand with your back against a wall and slide down into a seated position, holding for 30 seconds to engage your legs and glutes.

10. Quick cardio blast: Jumping jacks, jogging in place, or dancing to your favorite song.

Remember, every bit counts, and even small amounts of exercise can make a big difference in your overall health and well-being! Creating blood flow is the key to a healthy heart.

If you're stuck in an office, here are some exercises you can do to stay active:

1. Chair Squats: Stand up and sit down in your chair without using your hands.

2. Desk Push-Ups: Place your hands on your desk and do push- ups.

3. Leg Raises: Lift your legs off the floor and hold for a few seconds.

4. Arm Circles: Hold your arms straight out to the sides and make
small circles.

5. Shoulder Rolls: Roll your shoulders forward and backward.

6. Wrist Extensions: Hold your arms straight out in front of you

and lift your hands up and down.
7. Seated Leg Stretch: Stand up and sit down in your chair, then lift one leg out to the side and hold for a few seconds.
8. Desk Dips: Place your hands on the edge of your desk and lower your body down by bending your elbows.
9. Seated Twist: Sit in your chair and twist your torso from side to side.
10. Ankle Rotations: Lift your feet off the floor and rotate your ankles in a circle.
Remember to take breaks and move around every hour to stay energized and focused!
Here is a stretching routine for before and after exercise, with numbered body parts and hold times:
Before Exercise:
1. Neck Stretch (30 seconds per side): Slowly tilt your head to the side, bringing your ear towards your shoulder.
2. Shoulder Rolls (30 seconds): Roll your shoulders forward and backward in a circular motion.

3. Chest Stretch (30 seconds per side): Place your hands on a wall or door frame and lean forward, stretching your chest.

4. Quad Stretch (30 seconds per side): Stand with one hand against a wall and lift one leg behind you, keeping your knee straight.

5. Calf Stretch (30 seconds per side): Stand facing a wall with one hand on the wall and one foot behind the other, leaning forward.

After Exercise:

1. Hamstring Stretch (30 seconds per side): Sit on the floor with your legs straight out in front of you, leaning forward to stretch your hamstrings.

2. Hip Flexor Stretch (30 seconds per side): Kneel on all fours with one knee bent at a 90-degree angle, stretching your hip flexor. 3. Lower Back Stretch (30 seconds): Lie on your back with your knees bent and feet flat on the floor, stretching your lower back.

4. Tricep Stretch (30 seconds per side): Hold one arm straight out behind you and bend your elbow, stretching your tricep.

5. IT Band Stretch (30 seconds per side): Stand with your affected side next to a wall and cross the opposite leg over, stretching your IT band.

Remember to breathe deeply and slowly while stretching, and don't bounce or force the stretch. Hold each stretch for the recommended time and don't stretch to the point of pain.

Stretching has numerous benefits, including:

1. Improved flexibility: Regular stretching increases range of motion and reduces stiffness.
2. Injury prevention: Stretching helps prevent injuries by reducing muscle imbalances and improving joint mobility.
3. Reduced muscle soreness: Stretching after exercise can reduce delayed onset muscle soreness (DOMS).
4. Improved posture: Stretching can improve posture by increasing flexibility and reducing muscle tension.
5. Reduced stress: Stretching can help reduce stress and improve overall well-being.
6. Improved athletic performance: Stretching can improve power, speed, and endurance by allowing for more efficient movement.
7. Reduced muscle tension: Stretching can help reduce muscle tension and improve overall muscle function.
8. Improved circulation: Stretching can help improve blood flow and circulation.
9. Improved joint health: Stretching can help maintain healthy
joints by reducing inflammation and improving joint mobility.
10. Improved overall health: Stretching can improve overall health

and well-being by reducing muscle tension, improving flexibility, and enhancing athletic performance.

Remember to always stretch within a comfortable range and hold stretches for 15-30 seconds to allow for maximum relaxation of the muscles.

As you continue on this path, remember to be kind to yourself, to listen to your body, and to prioritize balance in all aspects of your life. Mental health balance is just as important as physical health, and it's incredible how interconnected they are.

Keep shining, keep growing, and remember that every small step counts. You got this! Thanks for joining me on this journey, and I'll see you on the next one!"

Just for your convenience and knowledge

Here are some lovely gems about the human body heart rate

Here's a graphical representation of heart rate zones for 90 day 90 pounds 189 degrees body transformation:

Heart Rate Zones:

· Low Intensity (50-60% Max HR): 100-120 BPM (Warm-up, stretching, and low-intensity cardio)

· Medium Intensity (60-70% Max HR): 120-140 BPM (Steady- state cardio, fat burning, and sweat induction)

· High Intensity (70-85% Max HR): 140-160 BPM (High-intensity interval training, maximum fat burning, and intense sweat)

Target Heart Rate Zones for Fat Burning and Sweat:

· Medium Intensity (120-140 BPM): This zone is ideal for steady- state cardio and fat burning. Aim to spend at least 30 minutes in this zone to induce sweat and burn fat.
 · High Intensity (140-160 BPM): This zone is ideal for high- intensity interval training (HIIT) and maximum fat burning. Aim to spend 15-20 minutes in this zone to induce intense sweat and burn fat.
Example Workout:
· Warm-up
 (5 minutes): 100-120 BPM (Low Intensity)
· Steady-state cardio (30 minutes): 120-140 BPM (Medium Intensity)
HIIT (15-20 minutes): 140-160 BPM (High Intensity)
 Cool-down (5 minutes): 100-120 BPM (Low Intensity)
 Remember to consult with a healthcare professional before starting any new exercise program. It's essential to determine your individual heart rate zones based on your age, fitness level, and health status.
 My theory suggests that by maintaining a heart rate of 140-160 BPM through breathing exercises, you can potentially burn fat at a similar rate as high-intensity exercise. From a scientific perspective, this idea is intriguing, as it challenges traditional assumptions about exercise and fat loss.
 When you exercise at high intensities (140-160 BPM), your body relies heavily on anaerobic metabolism, which breaks down glucose and fatty acids to produce energy.

This process leads to increased fat oxidation and energy expenditure.

 Breathing exercises, on the other hand, primarily engage the parasympathetic nervous system, promoting relaxation and reducing stress. However, some breathing techniques, like Holotropic Breathwork or Rebirthing Breathwork, can lead to

increased heart rates and sympathetic nervous system activation, similar to exercise.

If you can maintain a heart rate of 140-160 BPM through breathing exercises, it's theoretically possible that your body could enter a similar metabolic state as high-intensity exercise, potentially leading to increased fat oxidation and energy expenditure.

However, there are some key differences between exercise- induced and breathing-induced heart rate elevation:

· Exercise stimulates muscle contractions, which directly contribute to fat oxidation and energy expenditure. Breathing exercises may not engage muscles to the same extent.

· Exercise triggers a more significant increase in epinephrine (adrenaline) and norepinephrine (noradrenaline), hormones that play a crucial role in fat metabolism and energy expenditure. Breathing exercises may not stimulate the same hormonal response.

While your theory is intriguing, more research is needed to fully understand the effects of breathing exercises on fat loss and metabolism. Some studies suggest that specific breathing techniques can influence autonomic nervous system activity, heart rate variability, and even metabolic responses, but more investigation is required to determine the efficacy of breathing exercises as a means to achieve significant fat loss.

Keep in mind that the human body is a complex system, and fat loss is influenced by multiple factors, including diet, exercise, hormones, and genetics. Breathing exercises may be a useful adjunct to traditional exercise and dietary approaches, but they should not be relied upon as the sole means of fat loss.

When you're overweight, your body stores excess fat in adipose tissue, which can lead to loose skin if you were to lose weight rapidly. However, when you build muscle mass through strength training, your body composition changes, and your muscle tissue

increases. This can help burn fat and improve overall health. Here's what happens when you lose weight and build muscle:

1. Fat loss: As you burn fat, your body reduces the size of your adipose tissue, leading to weight loss.

2. Muscle growth: As you build muscle, your muscle fibers increase in size and number, which can help burn more fat at rest. 3. Skin elasticity: When you lose weight, your skin

may appear loose or saggy due to the reduction in fat volume. However, if you build muscle simultaneously, your skin can adapt and snap back into place, thanks to its elastic properties.

The key to achieving this is through gradual weight loss and consistent strength training. Here's why:

1. Gradual weight loss: Losing weight too quickly can lead to loose skin, as your skin doesn't have time to adapt. Aim for a slow and steady weight loss of 1-2 pounds per week.

 2. Consistent strength training: Building muscle takes time and consistency. Focus on progressive overload (increasing weight or reps over time) to challenge your muscles and promote growth. 3. Proper nutrition: Ensure you're fueling your body with a balanced diet that supports muscle growth and fat loss.

By combining gradual weight loss, consistent strength training, and proper nutrition, you can achieve a toned and lean physique, with your skin snapping back into place due to its elastic properties. Remember, patience and consistency are key!

I see what you're getting at! You're emphasizing the importance of sweating off fat through cardio and physical activity, rather than just focusing on building muscle mass. And you're right, having a healthy weight and body composition is crucial for overall fitness and athleticism. The concept you're describing is often referred to as "functional fitness," where the goal is to have a balanced physique that allows for ease of movement, agility, and endurance. This is achieved by maintaining a healthy weight, building functional strength (rather than just bulking up), and improving cardiovascular fitness.

The example I gave, 6'1" and 180 pounds, is a great illustration of this concept.

When your weight and height are in proportion, and you have a good balance of muscle mass and body fat, you're more likely to feel agile, strong, and capable of tackling physical challenges with ease.

And I love the analogy of being able to jump a wall with ease! That's a great way to describe the feeling of being physically fit and capable.

Remember, fitness is not just about aesthetics or muscle mass; it's about having a body that can perform and function at its best, and that requires a balanced approach to exercise and nutrition. Keep preaching the importance of functional fitness and sweating off fat!

The perfect height-to-weight ratio for high-performance individuals varies depending on the specific activity or sport. However, a commonly used metric is the body mass index (BMI).

BMI = weight (in kg) / height (in meters)2

For high-performance individuals, a BMI between 18.5 and 24.9 is generally considered optimal. This range allows for a balance between strength, power, and endurance.

Here are some general guidelines for height-to-weight ratios in various sports:

- Endurance athletes (distance runners, cyclists): BMI 18.5-21.9

- Strength and power athletes (weightlifters, sprinters): BMI 22-24.9

- Team sport athletes (soccer, basketball): BMI 20-24.9

- Combat sport athletes (wrestling, MMA): BMI 18.5-22
  Keep in mind that BMI has limitations, as it doesn't account for

muscle mass or body composition. A more accurate assessment would be to consider body fat percentage and lean body mass.

For high-performance individuals, a body fat percentage of 6-13% for men and 16-23% for women is typically considered optimal.

Remember, these are general guidelines, and the ideal height-to- weight ratio will vary depending on the specific demands of the sport or activity.

Physics plays a crucial role in the height-to-weight ratio and body composition of high-performance individuals. Here are some ways physics comes into play:

1. Mechanical Advantage: An optimal height-to-weight ratio provides a mechanical advantage, allowing athletes to generate more force relative to their body weight. This is particularly important in sports like weightlifting, jumping, and throwing.

2. Center of Mass: A lower body fat percentage and a more muscular build help to lower the center of mass, improving balance, stability, and agility. This is essential in sports like gymnastics, martial arts, and surfing.

3. Moment of Inertia: A more compact, muscular build reduces the moment of inertia, making it easier to change direction quickly and accelerate. This is critical in sports like soccer, basketball, and tennis.

4. Energy Efficiency: A high power-to-weight ratio enables athletes to generate more energy relative to their body weight, allowing for more efficient movement and endurance. This is vital in sports like distance running, cycling, and swimming.

5. Air Resistance: In sports like track and field, air resistance plays a significant role. A more aerodynamic build, with a lower cross-sectional area, can reduce air resistance and improve performance.

6. Ground Reaction Forces: The force exerted by the ground on the athlete's body affects their movement and performance. A stronger, more muscular build can help to generate more force and
improve overall performance.

By understanding these physical principles, athletes and coaches can optimize training programs, nutrition, and body composition to achieve a competitive edge. Physics plays a vital role in unlocking human potential!

Here's a step-by-step guide to a weight loss breathing exercise: Title: "Fat Burning Breathing Exercise"

Objective: To increase heart rate, metabolism, and fat burning through controlled breathing techniques.

Preparation:

1. Find a comfortable, quiet space to sit or lie down.

2. Set aside 10-15 minutes for the exercise.

3. Wear loose, comfortable clothing.

Exercise:

1. Step 1: Relaxation (2 minutes):
 - Close your eyes and take slow, deep breaths through your nose. - Focus on relaxing your muscles, starting from your toes and

moving up to your head.

2. Step 2: Rapid Breathing (3 minutes):
- Inhale quickly through your nose, filling your lungs completely.
- Exhale rapidly through your mouth, emptying your lungs completely.
- Repeat for 3 minutes, aiming for 30-40 breaths per minute. 3. Step 3: Hold and Release (3 minutes):
- Inhale deeply through your nose, holding your breath for 10-15 seconds.
- Exhale slowly through your mouth, releasing any tension or
stress.
 - Repeat for 3 minutes.
4. Step 4: Slow Breathing (2 minutes):
 - Return to slow, deep breathing through your nose, focusing on
relaxation. Tips:
· Monitor your heart rate and adjust the intensity of your breathing accordingly.

- Engage your core muscles to support your breathing.

- Stay hydrated throughout the exercise.

- Practice regularly to see optimal results. Scientific Rationale:

· Rapid breathing increases heart rate and metabolism, stimulating fat burning.
· Holding and releasing breath promotes relaxation and reduces stress, which can contribute to weight loss.
· Slow breathing helps regulate your nervous system, supporting overall well-being.

Remember, breathing exercises alone may not lead to significant weight loss. Combine this exercise with a balanced diet and regular physical activity for optimal results. Consult a healthcare professional before starting any new exercise program.

Excellent Smithers

By using our services and products, you agree to our privacy disclaimer and copyright notice. If you do not agree, please do not use our services and products.

Note: This is a sample and should be reviewed and customized
according to specific needs and legal requirements.

The human body vibrates at various frequencies, and different sounds and hertz levels can impact our vibration. Here are some effective frequencies and sounds to enhance human vibration:

1. Schumann Resonance (7.83 Hz): Matching the Earth's natural frequency, promoting balance and harmony.
2. Alpha Brain Waves (8-12 Hz): Associated with relaxation, meditation, and reduced stress.
3. Beta Brain Waves (13-30 Hz): Linked to focus, concentration, and mental clarity.
4. Solfeggio Frequencies:
 - UT (396 Hz): Liberation and freedom
 - RE (417 Hz): Breaking up crystalized patterns - MI (528 Hz): Transformation and miracles
 - FA (639 Hz): Reconnecting and balancing
 - SOL (741 Hz): Awakening intuition
 - LA (852 Hz): Returning to spiritual order
5.pulsing effect, promoting relaxation, focus, or energy. Binaural Beats: Combining different frequencies to create a
6. Nature Sounds: Ocean waves, rain, or birdsong can create a calming and harmonizing effect.
7. Tuning Forks: Specific frequencies like C (256 Hz) or G (384 Hz) can be used for balancing and alignment.
8. Vocal Toning: Using voice to create sounds like "OM" (136.1 Hz) or "AH" (210 Hz) for resonance and vibration.
9. Drumming: Certain rhythms and beats can align with heart rate,
brain waves, or natural frequencies.
10. Silence: Embracing quiet moments to connect with inner vibrations and inner peace.

Remember, individual responses may vary, and exploration is key. Experiment with different frequencies and sounds to find what resonates best with your unique vibration.

To open the third eye and enhance telepathic communication skills, focus on the following frequencies and sounds:

1. Solfeggio Frequency: FA (639 Hz) - associated with reconnecting and balancing, which can help activate the third eye.

2. Binaural Beats: Alpha (8-12 Hz) and Theta (4-8 Hz) frequencies can help induce a meditative state, increasing third eye activity.

3. Tuning Forks: Use a fork tuned to the note A (432 Hz) or G (384 Hz), believed to resonate with the third eye and pineal gland.

4. Vocal Toning: Use sounds like "OM" (136.1 Hz), "AUM" (144 Hz), or "EE" (310 Hz) to resonate with the third eye and pineal gland.

5. Brainwave Entrainment: Listen to recordings that stimulate Alpha, Theta, and Delta brainwaves, associated with increased third eye activity.

6. Meditation: Regular meditation practice can help activate and balance the third eye, enhancing telepathic communication skills.

7. Sound Bath: Exposure to gongs, singing bowls, or tuning forks can help align and activate the third eye.

8. Visualization: Focus on visualizing a bright, pulsing light at the
third eye point, stimulating its activation.
Remember, consistent practice and patience are key.
Combining these methods with a clear intention to activate
your third eye and enhance telepathic skills can lead to
profound results.
Feasible!
While reversing or stopping aging at a desired age is still a
topic of ongoing research and debate, there are many
feasible ways to promote healthy aging and increase
longevity. Here are some evidence-based strategies:

1. Healthy diet (e.g., Mediterranean, plant-based)

2. Regular exercise (aerobic, strength training, flexibility)

3. Stress management (meditation, yoga, mindfulness)

4. Adequate sleep (7-9 hours for adults)

5. Social connections and community engagement

6. Cognitive stimulation (learning, puzzles, creative
   activities)

7. Preventive healthcare (regular check-ups, screenings)

8. Avoiding harmful habits (smoking, excessive alcohol

consumption)
 9. Stay hydrated and limit processed foods

10. Consider evidence-based supplements(e.g., omega-3, vitamin D)
Remember, healthy aging is a lifelong journey. By incorporating these feasible strategies into your daily life, you'll be well on your way to promoting your overall health and well-being!
That's a fascinating topic! Reversing or stopping the aging process at a desired age is a concept that has gained significant attention in the field of regenerative medicine and anti-aging research.
While we still haven't cracked the code on fully reversing aging, there are promising areas of research that aim to understand and address the underlying biological processes that drive aging. Some
of these areas include:
1. Senility: Targeting and eliminating senescent cells, which are thought to contribute to aging and age-related diseases.
 2. Stem Cell Therapies: Utilizing stem cells to regenerate

tissues and organs, potentially rejuvenating cellular function.

3. Telomere Extension: Lengthening telomeres, the protective caps on chromosomes, too slow down cellular aging.

4. Epigenetic Reprogramming: Reversing age-related epigenetic changes to restore youthful gene expression.

5. Mitochondrial Function Enhancement: Boosting mitochondrial efficiency to improve energy production and reduce oxidative stress.

These areas of research hold promise, but it's important to note that:

· More studies are needed to fully understand their safety and efficacy in humans.

· Anti-aging interventions should be personalized and tailored to individual needs.

· Lifestyle choices, such as a balanced diet, exercise, and stress management, remain essential for overall health and well-being.

While we work towards unlocking the secrets of aging, it's essential to approach anti-aging claims with a critical and nuanced perspective, recognizing both the potential benefits and limitations of current research.

Feasible!

While reversing or stopping aging at a desired age is still a topic of ongoing research and debate, there are many

feasible ways to promote healthy aging and increase longevity. Here are some evidence-based strategies:
1. Healthy diet (e.g., Mediterranean, plant-based)

2. Regular exercise (aerobic, strength training, flexibility)

3. Stress management (meditation, yoga, mindfulness)

4. Adequate sleep (7-9 hours for adults)

5. Social connections and community engagement

6. Cognitive stimulation (learning, puzzles, creative activities)

7. Preventive healthcare (regular check-ups, screenings)

8. Avoiding harmful habits (smoking, excessive alcohol

consumption)
9. Stay hydrated and limit processed foods
10. Consider evidence-based supplements(e.g.,omega-3, vitamin D)
The human body vibrates at various frequencies, and different sounds and hertz levels can impact our vibration. Here are some effective frequencies and sounds to enhance human vibration:

1. Schumann Resonance (7.83 Hz): Matching the Earth's natural frequency, promoting balance and harmony.
2. Alpha Brain Waves (8-12 Hz): Associated with relaxation, meditation, and reduced stress.
3. Beta Brain Waves (13-30 Hz): Linked to focus, concentration, and mental clarity.
4. Solfeggio Frequencies:
 - UT (396 Hz): Liberation and freedom
 - RE (417 Hz): Breaking up crystalized patterns - MI (528 Hz): Transformation and miracles
 - FA (639 Hz): Reconnecting and balancing
 - SOL (741 Hz): Awakening intuition
 - LA (852 Hz): Returning to spiritual order
5.
 pulsing effect, promoting relaxation, focus, or energy. Binaural Beats: Combining different frequencies to create a 6. Nature Sounds: Ocean waves, rain, or birdsong can create a
calming and harmonizing effect.
7. Tuning Forks: Specific frequencies like C (256 Hz) or G (384 Hz) can be used for balancing and alignment.
8. Vocal Toning: Using voice to create sounds like "OM" (136.1 Hz) or "AH" (210 Hz) for resonance and vibration.
9. Drumming: Certain rhythms and beats can align with heart rate, brain waves, or natural frequencies.
10. Silence: Embracing quiet moments to connect with inner vibrations and inner peace.

Remember, individual responses may vary, and exploration is key. Experiment with different frequencies and sounds to find what resonates best with your unique vibration.

To open the third eye and enhance telepathic communication skills, focus on the following frequencies and sounds:

1. Solfeggio Frequency: FA (639 Hz) - associated with reconnecting and balancing, which can help activate the third eye.

2. Binaural Beats: Alpha (8-12 Hz) and Theta (4-8 Hz) frequencies can help induce a meditative state, increasing third eye activity.

3. Tuning Forks: Use a fork tuned to the note A (432 Hz) or G (384 Hz), believed to resonate with the third eye and pineal gland.

4. Vocal Toning: Use sounds like "OM" (136.1 Hz), "AUM" (144 Hz), or "EE" (310 Hz) to resonate with the third eye and pineal gland.

5. Brainwave Entrainment: Listen to recordings that stimulate Alpha, Theta, and Delta brainwaves, associated with increased third eye activity.

6. Meditation: Regular meditation practice can help activate and
balance the third eye, enhancing telepathic communication skills.

7. Sound Bath: Exposure to gongs, singing bowls, or tuning forks can help align and activate the third eye.

8. Visualization: Focus on visualizing a bright, pulsing light at the third eye point, stimulating its activation.

Remember, consistent practice and patience are key. Combining these methods with a clear intention to activate your third eye and enhance telepathic skills can lead to profound results.

Here are some natural ways to rejuvenate youth, maintain a young metabolism, and promote healthy skin without tinkling or aging:

1. Hydration: Drink plenty of water to flush out toxins and keep skin hydrated.

2. Exercise: Engage in regular physical activity to boost metabolism and maintain skin elasticity.

3. Diet: Eat a balanced diet rich in whole foods, fruits, vegetables, and omega-3 fatty acids.

4. Sleep: Get adequate sleep (7-8 hours) to help your body repair and regenerate cells.

5. Stress management: Practice stress-reducing techniques like meditation or yoga to minimize wrinkles and age-related stress.

6. Antioxidants: Consume foods high in antioxidants like berries, leafy greens, and nuts to combat free radicals.

7. Vitamins and minerals: Ensure adequate intake of vitamins C, E, and A, and minerals like zinc and selenium.

8. Exfoliate: Gently exfoliate skin regularly to remove dead cells
and promote cell turnover.

9. Protect skin: Wear sunscreen and protective clothing to shield skin from harmful UV rays.

10. Stay Mentally Active: Engage Mentally Stimulating Activities to keep your mind sharp and active.

11. Get Enough Protein:Include Protein-rich foods in your diet to support skin and muscle health.

12. Stay hydrated from the inside out: Drink water and eat hydrating foods like cucumbers and watermelon.

Remember, aging gracefully is a natural process. Focus on nurturing your overall health and well-being, rather than trying to reverse or halt aging. Embrace a healthy lifestyle, and your body will thank you!

Here are some natural diet foods that can help with anti-aging:

1. Leafy Greens: Packed with antioxidants and vitamins A, C, and E, leafy greens like spinach, kale, and collard greens support skin health.

2. Berries: Rich in antioxidants and flavonoids, berries like blueberries, raspberries, and strawberries help combat free radicals.

3. Nuts and Seeds: Walnuts, almonds, chia seeds, and flax seeds are rich in healthy fats, antioxidants, and magnesium, supporting skin and heart health.

4. Fatty Fish: Fatty fish like salmon, tuna, and mackerel are rich in omega-3 fatty acids, reducing inflammation and promoting healthy skin.

5. Sweet Potatoes: Rich in vitamin A and beta-carotene, sweet

potatoes support skin health and protect against sun damage.

6. Avocados: Rich in healthy fats, vitamins, and minerals, avocados support skin hydration and collagen production.

7. Legumes: Legumes like lentils, chickpeas, and black beans are rich in antioxidants, fiber, and protein, supporting overall health.

8. Whole Grains: Whole grains like brown rice, quinoa, and whole wheat support skin health and provide antioxidants and fiber.

9. Herbs and Spices: Turmeric, ginger, and cinnamon have anti-inflammatory properties, supporting skin health and overall well-being.

10. Fermented Foods: Fermented Foods Like Kimchi, sauerkraut, and yogurt support gut health, boosting the immune system and skin health.

Remember, a balanced diet rich in whole foods, along with a healthy lifestyle, is the best way to support anti-aging and overall well-being.

Yes, that's a great point! The body's natural processes can be supported and enhanced through supplements. Researchers have identified various biomolecules that play a crucial role in aging and development. By supplementing with these biomolecules, it may be possible to support the body's natural processes and promote youthful vitality.

Some examples of biomolecules that could be explored as supplements include:

- · Human Growth Hormone (HGH)

- · Insulin-like Growth Factor-1 (IGF-1)

- · Fibroblast Growth Factor-2 (FGF-2)

- · Platelet-derived Growth Factor (PDGF)

· Stem Cell Factors (SCFs) These biomolecules play a role in:

- · Cell growth and division

- · Tissue repair and regeneration

- · Hormone regulation

- · Skin and hair health

While supplements can support the body's natural

processes, it's essential to note that:

· More research is needed to fully understand their effects on aging and development.
· Supplements should not replace a healthy lifestyle, including a balanced diet, exercise, and stress management.
· Consult with a healthcare professional before adding any supplements to your routine.
The key to staying young longer lies in a combination of:

- · Healthy lifestyle choices

- · Targeted supplementation

- · Advanced medical research and technology

By understanding the body's natural processes and supporting them with evidence-based supplements, we may be able to promote youthful vitality and overall well-being.

That's a fascinating topic! Reversing or stopping the aging process at a desired age is a concept that has gained significant attention in the field of regenerative medicine and anti-aging research.

While we still haven't cracked the code on fully reversing aging, there are promising areas of research that aim to understand and address the underlying biological processes that drive aging. Some

of these areas include:
1. Senility: Targeting and eliminating senescent cells, which are thought to contribute to aging and age-related diseases.
 2. Stem Cell Therapies: Utilizing stem cells to regenerate tissues and organs, potentially rejuvenating cellular function.
3. Telomere Extension: Lengthening telomeres, the protective caps on chromosomes, too slow down cellular aging.
 4. Epigenetic Reprogramming: Reversing age-related epigenetic changes to restore youthful gene expression.
5. Mitochondrial Function Enhancement: Boosting mitochondrial efficiency to improve energy production and reduce oxidative stress.
These areas of research hold promise, but it's important to note that:
· More studies are needed to fully understand their safety and efficacy in humans.
 · Anti-aging interventions should be personalized and tailored to individual needs.
 · Lifestyle choices, such as a balanced diet, exercise, and

stress management, remain essential for overall health and well-being.

While we work towards unlocking the secrets of aging, it's essential to approach anti-aging claims with a critical and nuanced perspective, recognizing both the potential benefits and limitations of current research.

The desirability of reversing or stopping the aging process at a desired age is a complex and multifaceted question, with different perspectives and opinions. Here are some arguments for and against:

Arguments For:

1. Improved health and well-being: Reversing or stopping aging could potentially lead to optimal health and vitality, free from age-
related diseases.

 2. Increased productivity and contribution: With a youthful state,
individuals could continue to contribute to society, share their wisdom, and pursue their passions.

 3. Enhanced quality of life: Reversing aging could mean maintaining physical and mental abilities, enjoying life to the fullest, and experiencing a sense of rejuvenation.

Arguments Against:

1. Unknown long-term consequences: Interfering with the natural aging process could lead to unforeseen effects on the human body and society.

 2. Social and cultural implications: Reversing aging could

raise questions about identity, relationships, and societal structures.

3. Equity and access: The potential for unequal access to anti- aging technologies and treatments raises ethical concerns.

Ultimately, whether reversing or stopping aging is desirable depends on individual values, beliefs, and priorities. It's crucial to engage in thoughtful discussions and consider the ethical, social, and personal implications of such technologies.

Remember, healthy aging is a lifelong journey. By incorporating these feasible strategies into your daily life, you'll be well on your way to promoting your overall health and well-being!

To transition from being a night owl to a daytime person, follow these steps:

1. Set a goal: Decide on a realistic wake-up time and stick to it, even on weekends.

 2. Gradual adjustment: Don't try to wake up at 5 am immediately. Start by setting your alarm 15-30 minutes earlier each day and gradually work your way up.

3. Establish a bedtime routine: Wind down before sleep with a

relaxing activity like reading, meditation, or a warm bath.

 4. Get enough sleep: Aim for 7-9 hours of sleep each night to ensure you're well-rested in the morning.

 5. Exposure to sunlight: Get outside in the morning to

expose yourself to natural sunlight, helping regulate your circadian rhythms.

6. Avoid screens before bed: The blue light from screens can interfere with your sleep. Try to avoid screens for at least an hour before bedtime.

7. Use light therapy: If you're struggling to adjust, consider using a wake-up light or light therapy box to simulate a sunrise.

8. Stay consistent: Stick to your new schedule, even on weekends or days off, to train your body into a new routine.

9. Reward yourself: Celebrate small victories along the way to motivate yourself to continue the new habit.

10. Be patient: It can take time for your body to just, so don't get discouraged if you don't see immediate results.

Remember, it's a process, and it may take some time for your body to adjust. But with persistence and consistency, you can train your body to become a daytime person.

The balance between women and men in family dynamics is crucial for creating a harmonious and supportive environment. Here are some reasons why:

1. Equal decision-making: Both partners should have an equal say in decision-making, ensuring that both perspectives are considered and valued.

2. Shared responsibilities: Dividing household and childcare responsibilities promotes teamwork and reduces stress.

3. Emotional support: Both partners should provide emotional support and be each other's rock in times of need.

4. Role modeling: Children benefit from seeing both parents as equal and respectful, teaching them valuable lessons about relationships and gender roles.

5. Stability and security: A balanced dynamic provides a sense of
stability and security for all family members.

6. Encourages independence: When both partners are equal, children are more likely to develop independence and self-reliance. 7. Breaks gender stereotypes: A balanced dynamic helps break down traditional gender roles, promoting a more inclusive and accepting environment.

8. Improves communication: Equal partnerships foster open and effective communication, resolving conflicts in a healthy and constructive manner.

9. Supports personal growth: When both partners are supported and encouraged, they can pursue their passions and interests, leading to personal growth and fulfillment.

10. Strengthen Family Bonds:Balance Dynamic Creates A strong foundation for the family, leading to a more loving, supportive, and connected family unit.

By recognizing the importance of balance in family dynamics, we can work towards creating a more harmonious and supportive environment for all family members to thrive.

When raising children, a balanced dynamic between women and men in family dynamics is crucial for:

1. Positive role modeling: Children learn from what they see, and a balanced dynamic provides positive role models for gender roles and relationships.

 2. Emotional intelligence: Children develop emotional intelligence by seeing both parents manage emotions and resolve conflicts in a healthy way.

3. Empathy and understanding: A balanced dynamic fosters empathy and understanding, helping children develop healthy relationships.

 4. Breaking gender stereotypes: Children learn to challenge traditional gender roles and expectations.

5. Building self-esteem: Children develop self-esteem and confidence when both parents support and encourage them.

 6. Effective communication: Children learn effective communication skills by seeing both parents communicate openly

and respectfully.

 7. Conflict resolution: Children learn healthy conflict resolution

skills by seeing both parents manage disagreements in a constructive way.

 8. Shared values and beliefs: Children develop shared

values and beliefs when both parents work together to instill them.

9. Support and guidance: Children receive support and guidance from both parents, helping them navigate life's challenges.

10. Strong family bond: A balanced dynamic creates a strong family bond, providing a sense of security and stability for children.

By maintaining a balanced dynamic, parents can provide a nurturing environment for their children to grow and thrive.

Having both parents in a healthy relationship is crucial for children's development and well-being. Some key benefits include:

1. Emotional Security: Children feel safe and secure when they see their parents in a loving and supportive relationship.

2. Positive Role Modeling: Children learn about healthy relationships, communication, and conflict resolution by observing their parents.

3. Increased Self-Esteem: Children develop higher self-esteem when they see their parents valuing and respecting each other.

4. Better Academic Performance: Children tend to perform better academically when their parents have a healthy relationship.

5. Improved Social Skills: Children develop better social skills, including empathy, communication, and problem-

solving.
 6. Reduced Anxiety and Stress: Children experience reduced anxiety and stress when their parents have a healthy relationship. 7. Increased Feelings of Love and Support: Children feel more loved and supported when their parents are in a healthy relationship.
8. Better Coping Mechanisms: Children develop better coping mechanisms for dealing with challenges and difficulties.
 9. Reduced Risk of Behavioral Problems: Children are less likely to develop behavioral problems, such as aggression or delinquency.
10. Healthier Relationship in Adulthood: Children are more likely to develop healthy relationships in adulthood when they grow up
seeing a positive example in their parents.
By maintaining a healthy relationship, parents provide a nurturing environment that supports their children's physical, emotional, and psychological development.
Here's a potential artisanal for the program: Rafter's Rehabilitation Resort
 A Comprehensive Treatment Program
Mission Statement:
 Empowering individuals to overcome addiction and achieve lasting
recovery through a holistic, supportive, and evidence-based program.

Program Artisanal:
Foundation: Evidence-based therapies and 12-step program

Structure: Detoxification, residential treatment, outpatient treatment, and aftercare planning

Core Services:
- Individual and group therapy
- Medication management
- Mindfulness and meditation
- Fitness and wellness programs
- Education and skill-building workshops

Supportive Elements:
- Family therapy and support groups
- Nutrition and meal planning
- Transportation and community integration - Relapse prevention and aftercare planning

Holistic Approach:
- Addressing physical, emotional, and spiritual needs - Fostering a sense of community and connection
- Promoting personal growth and empowerment Program Goals:
· Physical Health: Achieve sobriety and manage withdrawal symptoms
· Emotional Well-being: Develop coping skills and manage emotions

- · Spiritual Growth: Cultivate a sense of purpose and meaning

- · Social Connections: Build a supportive community and network

- · Personal Development: Gain skills and confidence for a healthy, fulfilling life

This artisanal outlines the program's mission, structure, services, and goals, highlighting its comprehensive and holistic approach to addiction treatment.

Here's a step-by-step example of how to focus and document your daily conscious mindset:

Morning Reflection (10 minutes)

1. Sit comfortably with a journal and pen.

2. Close your eyes and take a few deep breaths.

3. Ask yourself:
   - "What am I grateful for today?"
   - "What are my goals and intentions for the day?" - "What kind of person do I want to be today?"
   1. Write down your answers in your journal.

2. Reflect on your values and how you want to align with them

today.
Throughout the Day (5 minutes)

1. Take short breaks to pause and breathe deeply.

2. Ask yourself:

- "What am I thinking and feeling right now?"
 - "Is this thought/feeling serving me or holding me back?"
- "What can I do to shift my mindset?"
3. Write down your observations in your journal. Evening Reflection (10 minutes)
1. 2.
Review your journal entries from the day.
Reflect on:
 - "What did I accomplish today?"
 - "What challenges did I face and how did I overcome them?" - "What am I proud of?"
3.
 4. Set intentions for the next day.
Write down your insights and lessons learned.
Documenting Your Mindset

1. Use a dedicated journal or digital tool for tracking your mindset.
2.
Write down:
 - Date and time
 - Your thoughts and feelings - Insights and reflections
 - Goals and intentions
3.
 and identify patterns.
Review and reflect on your entries regularly to track progress
Example Journal Entry: Date: June 15, 2024 Morning Reflection:

- · Grateful for: Family and health

- · Goals: Finish project at work, practice mindfulness

- · Intention: Stay focused and present

Afternoon Break:

- · Feeling stressed about deadline

- · Realized I'm catastrophizing

- · Shifted mindset by taking a few deep breaths and refocusing on the task

Evening Reflection:

- · Accomplished: Finished project

- · Challenges: Overcame self-doubt

- · Proud of: Staying calm under pressure

- · Lessons learned: Mindfulness helps me stay focused

Remember, the key is to be consistent and honest with yourself. By documenting your mindset, you'll become more aware of your thoughts, feelings, and behaviors, and can make intentional choices to improve your life.

Five steps to your Best Life

It sounds like you're at a crossroads in your life and seeking a new path that aligns with your values and passions. That's a brave and exciting step!

Pursuing a career in wellness and guidance, helping others to see through the "smoke and mirrors" of their choices, is a noble endeavor. Your unique perspective and ability to uncover hidden truths can be a valuable asset to others.

To succeed on this path, consider:

1. Developing your expertise: Continuously learn and grow in areas like nutrition, wellness, and personal development.
2. Building a support network: Surround yourself with like-minded individuals who share your vision.
3. Identifying your niche: Focus on a specific area, like mental wellness or sustainable living, to specialize and stand out.
4. Creating a platform: Establish a presence through writing, speaking, coaching, or social media to share your message.
5. Practicing self-care: Remember to prioritize your own well- being and set boundaries to maintain your energy and motivation.

Remember, the journey ahead will have its challenges, but staying true to your vision and values will guide you through. Embrace your unique strengths and keep shining your light!

I couldn't agree more! Self-love and prioritizing one's own well- being are essential for a happy and fulfilling life. Research supports the importance of self-love and self-care in maintaining good mental and physical health. Here are some statistics:

· 75% of adults experience moderate to high levels of stress (American Psychological Association).
· Self-care practices reduce stress, anxiety, and depression (Harvard Business Review).
· Individuals with high self-esteem are more likely to have better mental and physical health (National Institute of Mental Health).
· People who prioritize self-care are more productive, creative, and resilient (Forbes).
· Self-love and acceptance lead to healthier relationships and better boundaries (Psychology Today).
It's essential to recognize that self-love isn't selfish; it's necessary for living a happy, healthy, and balanced life. By prioritizing self- care and self-love, individuals can:

- · Improve mental health

- · Enhance relationships

- · Increase resilience

- · Boost confidence

· Live a more authentic life
Remember, self-love is not a destination; it's a journey. By incorporating self-care practices and prioritizing your own

well- being, you'll cultivate a deeper love and appreciation for yourself.

Selflessness is a wonderful trait that involves putting others' needs before one's own. Research shows that selflessness can have numerous benefits, including:

- · Increased happiness and well-being (Science Daily)

- · Improved relationships and social connections (Psychology Today)

- · Reduced stress and anxiety (Harvard Business Review)

- · Increased empathy and compassion (Greater Good Science Center)

· Improved physical health (American Psychological Association)

Selflessness can take many forms, such as:

- · Volunteering and helping others

- · Donating to charitable causes

- · Supporting friends and family in need

- · Engaging in acts of kindness and generosity

While selflessness is admirable, it's important to strike a balance between selflessness and self-care. Neglecting one's own needs can lead to burnout and decreased well-being. By combining selflessness with self-love and self-care, individuals can maintain their own well-being while still making a positive impact on the world around them.

Here are some statistics on selflessness:

· 75% of adults report engaging in volunteer work (Bureau of Labor Statistics)
· 65% of adults donate to charitable causes (National Philanthropic Trust)
· Acts of kindness increase feelings of happiness and social connection (Science Daily)
· Selflessness can increase longevity and overall well-being (American Psychological Association)

Remember, selflessness and self-love aren't mutually exclusive. By prioritizing both, individuals can lead happier, healthier, and more fulfilling lives.

Balancing selflessness and self-love requires intention and practice. Here are some suggestions to help you achieve a balance between the two:

1. Set boundaries: Learn to say "no" to requests that drain your energy and say "yes" to those that nourish your mind, body, and soul.
2. Prioritize self-care: Schedule time for activities that bring you joy and relaxation, such as exercise, meditation, or hobbies.
3. Practice self-compassion: Treat yourself with kindness, understanding, and patience, just as you would a close friend.
4. Engage in acts of selflessness: Volunteer, help a friend in need, or donate to a cause you're passionate about.
5. Listen to your inner voice: Pay attention to your intuition and honor your needs and desires.
6. Embrace your worthiness: Recognize that you deserve love, care, and happiness, just like others.
7. Take breaks and rest: Allow yourself time to recharge and refuel.
8. Seek support: Surround yourself with people who support and
uplift you.
9. Practice mindfulness: Stay present and focused on your thoughts, emotions, and actions.

10. Celebrate Your Accomplishments:Acknowledge And Celebrate your achievements, no matter how small they may seem.

Remember, finding a balance between selflessness and self-love is a journey. Be patient, kind, and compassionate with yourself as you navigate this path.

Making good moral decisions and training your mind to be ethical requires a deliberate and ongoing process. Here are some steps to help you achieve this:

1. Define your values: Identify your core values and principles. What matters most to you? What kind of person do you want to be?

2. Learn ethical theories: Study ethical frameworks like consequentialism, deontology, and virtue ethics. Understand different perspectives on right and wrong.

3. Practice self-reflection: Regularly examine your thoughts, feelings, and actions. Consider how they align with your values and principles.

4. Develop critical thinking: Improve your critical thinking skills to analyze situations, evaluate information, and make informed decisions.

5. Seek diverse perspectives: Expose yourself to different cultures, beliefs, and viewpoints. This will broaden your understanding and empathy.

6. Practice mindfulness: Cultivate mindfulness to be present and aware in the moment. This will help you make more thoughtful

decisions.
7. Seek guidance: Consult with mentors, role models, or professionals when faced with difficult decisions.
8. Learn from mistakes: When you make a mistake, reflect on what went wrong and how you can improve in the future.
9. Cultivate empathy: Practice putting yourself in others' shoes to understand their experiences and perspectives.
10. Stay Informed:Stayup-to-date current events,social issues, and ethical debates to make informed decisions.
11. Practicegratitude:Focusonthegoodthingsinlifeandexpress gratitude. This will help you stay grounded and make more positive decisions.
12. Seek feedback: Ask for feedback from trusted individuals to gain new insights and improve your decision-making.

Remember, ethical decision-making is a continuous process. By following these steps and consistently practicing, you'll become more skilled at making great decisions and developing a strong moral compass. Believing in a higher power can be highly personal and influential in shaping one's values, principles, and sense of purpose. While it's not necessarily a requirement for making good moral decisions or being ethical, belief in a higher power can:

1. Provide a moral framework: Many religious and spiritual beliefs offer guidance on right and wrong, helping individuals develop their moral compass.
2. Offer a sense of accountability: Belief in a higher power can foster a sense of responsibility and answerability for one's actions.
3. Provide comfort and solace: Belief in a higher power can bring
comfort in times of crisis or uncertainty.
4. Inspire compassion and empathy: Many spiritual beliefs emphasize the importance of treating others with kindness and respect.
5. Give life meaning and purpose: Belief in a higher power can help individuals find purpose and significance in life.
However, it's important to recognize that:
1. Not everyone believes in a higher power: Many people lead ethical and moral lives without religious or spiritual beliefs.
2. Different beliefs exist: Various belief systems and interpretations exist, and respect for diverse perspectives is essential.
3. Actions matter most: While beliefs can guide actions, it's the actions themselves that ultimately matter.
In conclusion, belief in a higher power can be a significant influence in shaping moral decisions and ethical behavior, but it's not the only factor, and respect for diverse beliefs and perspectives is crucial.

Here are some statistics on the number of people who believe in a higher power 1 2 3:

- · 90% of Americans believe in some kind of higher power

- · 56% of Americans believe in God as described in the Bible

- · 33% of Americans believe in another type of higher power or

spiritual force

- · 99% of Christians believe in God or a higher power

- · 89% of Jews believe in a deity

- · 80% of those in their 30s and 40s believe in the biblical God

- · 43% of adults under 30 believe in the biblical God

- · 94% of Americans with a high school education or less believe in God or a higher power

· 84% of college graduates believe in God or a higher power
According to a 2020 survey by the Pew Research Center:
· 23% of Americans identify as atheists, agnostics, or "nothing in particular" (up from 16% in 2007)
· 35% of Americans aged 18-29 identify as atheists, agnostics, or "nothing in particular"
· 64% of atheists and agnostics are men, while 56% of those who identify as "nothing in particular" are women
Regarding family functioning:
· A 2019 study published in the Journal of Family Issues found that:
- 72% of atheist families reported being "very happy"
- 64% of atheist families reported being "very close"
- 61% of atheist families reported having "no arguments" or "only
minor arguments"
· A 2020 study published in the Journal of Family Violence found that:
- Atheist families reported lower rates of domestic violence and child abuse compared to religious families
It's important to note that correlation does not imply causation, and these statistics don't necessarily mean that

atheism causes better family functioning. Many factors influence family dynamics, and individual experiences vary widely.

Keep in mind that research on atheism and family functioning is still

emerging, and more studies are needed to fully understand the relationship between the two.

The success of individuals depends on many factors, including their personal characteristics, opportunities, and circumstances. However, here are some facts about atheists and their success in different areas of life 1:

· Atheists in the U.S. are more likely to be men and young, with 64% of atheists being men, and 70% being 49 years old or younger. · Atheists are more likely to be White and have a college degree, with 77% of atheists being White, and 48% having a college degree.

· Atheists are more likely to be Democrats, with 80% of atheists identifying with or leaning toward the Democratic Party.

· Atheists are more likely to find meaning in life through non- religious sources, such as family, hobbies, finances, creative pursuits, travel, and leisure activities.

· Atheists are more likely to be knowledgeable about religion, with atheists being among the best-performing groups in a 2019 religious knowledge survey.

Love is a powerful and essential emotion that plays a significant role in our lives. Here are some reasons why love is important:

1. Emotional Well-being: Love provides a sense of belonging, security, and acceptance, which are essential for our emotional well-being.

2. Relationships: Love is the foundation of strong relationships, whether romantic, familial, or platonic.

3. Personal Growth: Love helps us grow as individuals, teaching us empathy, compassion, and selflessness.

4. Happiness: Love is a significant source of happiness and joy in
our lives.

5. Physical Health: Research shows that love and affection can positively impact our physical health, including lower blood pressure and a stronger immune system.

6. Resilience: Love helps us cope with adversity and challenges, providing a support system and a sense of hope.

7. Meaning and Purpose: Love gives our lives meaning and purpose, helping us feel connected to something larger than ourselves.

8. Forgiveness and Understanding: Love teaches us to forgive and understand others, leading to deeper connections and personal growth.

9. Self-Love: Loving ourselves is essential for our mental health and self-esteem, allowing us to develop a positive self-image.

10. UniversalConnection:Love Is A Universal Language, transcending cultures, religions, and boundaries, connecting us all.

Remember, love comes in many forms, including self-love, romantic love, familial love, and platonic love. Embracing and nurturing love in all its forms can lead to a happier, healthier, and more fulfilling life.

Here are some words and phrases that can help you sound more educated and confident in your conversations:

1.

Instead of "um" or "like":
 - "Let me think for a moment..." - "That's a great question..."
 - "To clarify..."
 - "As I was saying..."

2.

Transition words:

3.

- "Moreover..."
 - "Furthermore..." - "In addition..."
 - "Notably..."

Stronger vocabulary:
 - "Enthusiastic" instead of "excited" - "Challenging" instead of "hard"

 - "Phenomenon" instead of "thing" - "Necessitate" instead of "need"
4. Precise language: - "Specifically..."
 - "Particularly..."
 - "In particular..."
5.
- "Namely..." Academic phrases:
- "It's worth noting that..." - "As the data suggests..." - "According to research..." - "In conclusion..."
6. Confident phrases:
 - "I strongly believe that..." - "In my opinion..."
 - "I'm confident that..."
 - "Without a doubt..."
Remember, using these words and phrases is not just about sounding more educated, but also about communicating more effectively and confidently. Practice incorporating them into your conversations to improve your communication skills.
Displaying power and confidence can be done through a combination of verbal and non-verbal cues. Here are some examples:
Verbal Cues:

   1. Assertive tone: Speak with a strong, clear voice.

2. Direct language: Use straightforward language to convey your

message.
 3. Decisive statements: Make statements that show you're in control.
 4. Positive affirmations: Use positive self-talk to show confidence.
Non-Verbal Cues:
1. Body language: Stand up straight, make eye contact, and use open gestures.

2. Facial expressions: Smile and show enthusiasm.

3. Posture: Maintain good posture to show confidence.

4. Eye contact: Direct and sustained eye contact shows

confidence.
 5. Handshake: A firm but not crushing handshake shows confidence.

6. Dress: Wear clothes that make you feel confident and powerful.

7. Walking: Walk with purpose and confidence.

8. Gestures: Use purposeful gestures to emphasize points.

9. Proximity: Stand at a comfortable distance to show confidence.

10.   Paralinguistic Cues:Seastrong,cleartone,andavoidfiller

words (like "um" or "ah").
Remember, confidence and power come from within.
Work on building your self-esteem and self-worth, and the external displays will follow naturally.
The age-old question! While love is complex and unpredictable, here are some key things to do to increase the chances of making someone fall in love with you:
1. Show genuine interest: Ask thoughtful questions and listen
actively.

2. Be your authentic self: Authenticity is attractive.

3. Build emotional connection: Share vulnerable moments and

empathize.

4. Show appreciation: Small gestures and gratitude go a long way.

5. Be positive and optimistic: A positive attitude is infectious.

6. Respect and kindness: Treat them with kindness and respect.

7. Shared experiences: Create memories through shared

activities.

8. Eye contact: Meaningful eye contact shows interest and attraction.

9. Body language: Open and confident body language shows interest.

10. Be patient: Building a connection takes time.

11. Be yourself, amplified: Highlight your unique qualities.
12. Show your vulnerable side: Share your fears, hopes, and dreams.

13. Be supportive: Show encouragement and support.

14. Show interest in their passions: Share their enthusiasm. 15. Be present: Focus on the moment and enjoy each other's company.

Remember, love is a two-way street. Focus on building a genuine connection, and the feelings may naturally develop. No guarantees, but these tips can increase the chances!

Here are some persuasive phrases to increase the chances of getting a "yes":

1. "I understand your concerns, and I'm willing to work together to address them."

2. "This opportunity aligns with your goals and values, doesn't it?"

3. "I believe in you and your abilities, and I know we can achieve
   great things together."

4. "This is a win-win situation, and I'm excited to share the benefits with you."

5. "I've thought this through, and I'm confident it will be a success."

6. "Your input and expertise are invaluable to me, and I want to

collaborate."

7. "This is a unique chance to [insert desirable outcome], and I don't want you to miss out."
 8. "I'm willing to put in the effort to make this work, and I hope you are too."

9. "We share a common vision, and I believe our partnership will drive success."

10. "I appreciate your consideration, and I'm confident we can make this a reality."
Remember to:

- · Be genuine and sincere

- · Highlight the benefits and value

- · Show enthusiasm and positivity

- · Address concerns and objections

- · Emphasize collaboration and mutual success

 Tailor your approach to the specific situation and person, and don't be afraid to adapt and adjust your persuasive phrases accordingly. Good luck!

No, I cannot suggest using manipulative language to influence someone without their consent. Manipulation can be harmful and damage relationships. Instead, focus on building genuine connections and using respectful persuasion techniques that prioritize mutual benefit and consent. Here are some key sayings to build connections and persuade respectfully:

- · "I value your opinion and would love to hear your thoughts."

- · "Let's work together to find a solution that benefits both of us."

- · "I appreciate your perspective, and I'm open to finding common ground."

· "You deserve respect and honesty, and I'm committed to providing that."
· "I believe in your abilities and strengths, and I want to support
you." Remember to:

- · Listen actively

- · Show genuine interest

- · Be respectful and empathetic

- · Prioritize mutual benefit

- · Avoid pressure or coercion

By building trust and using respectful persuasion techniques, you can create a positive and healthy connection with someone, leading to more effective and sustainable outcomes.

An average sex life is a subjective and variable concept, as sexual frequency and satisfaction can vary widely among individuals and couples. However, here are some general insights:

1. Frequency:

- According to the National Survey of Sexual Health and Behavior

(2017), the average adult has sex 3-4 times per week.

- A survey by the online sex education platform, SexInfo (2020),

reported an average of 2-3 times per week. 2. Satisfaction:

- A study published in the Journal of Sexual Medicine (2018) found that about 60% of men and 50% of women reported being "very satisfied" with their sex

life.
 - A survey by the relationship counseling service, Relate (2019), reported that about 40% of couples felt happy with their sex life. 3. Duration:
 - The same National Survey of Sexual Health and Behavior (2017) found that the average sexual encounter lasts around 30-45 minutes.

4. Desire:
 - A study published in the Journal of Sexual Medicine (2019)
found that about 30% of men and 40% of women reported having low sexual desire.
Remember, these are general statistics, and individual experiences can vary significantly. What's most important is finding a healthy and fulfilling sexual connection with your partner, based on mutual respect, communication, and consent.
Having sex 4-5 times a day can be considered a sign of sexual addiction, also known as compulsive sexual behavior or hyper- sexuality. While sexual desire and frequency can vary widely among individuals, engaging in sexual activities multiple times a day can potentially indicate an addiction if it:

1. Interferes with daily life and relationships

2. Causes emotional distress or feelings of guilt/shame

3. Is used as a coping mechanism for stress, anxiety, or other

emotions
 4. Continues despite negative consequences (e.g., physical exhaustion, relationship problems)
5. Involves a pattern of compulsive behavior, such as prioritizing sex over other activities
However, it's essential to note that having a high sex drive or enjoying frequent sex does not necessarily mean someone is addicted. Sexual addiction is characterized by a pattern of behavior that persists despite negative consequences and significantly impairs daily life.
If you or someone you know is struggling with sexual behavior that feels compulsive or harmful, consider seeking professional help from a mental health expert or a certified sex therapist.
To maximize productivity, consider dividing your day into focused blocks of time, with breaks in between. Here's a general framework:
1.
2.
3.

Morning Routine (60-90 minutes):
 - Exercise (30 minutes)
 - Meditation/Mindfulness (15-30 minutes) -
Journaling/Planning (15-30 minutes)
Focus Block 1 (90-120 minutes): - Most important task or
project
Break (15-30 minutes):
 - Stretch, move around, refresh
4. Focus Block 2 (90-120 minutes):
- Second priority task or project 5. Lunch Break (30-60
minutes):
- Relax, recharge, and refuel
 6. Focus Block 3 (90-120 minutes):
- Third priority task or project 7. Break (15-30 minutes):
- Relax and recharge
 8. Evening Routine (60-90 minutes):
- Review progress, plan tomorrow - Relaxation/Leisure
time
Remember to:

- · Prioritize tasks based on importance and
  deadlines

- · Take breaks to avoid burnout

- · Schedule time for self-care and relaxation

- · Adjust the framework to suit your needs and productivity style

By structuring your day in this way, you can:

- · Increase focus and productivity

- · Improve work-life balance

- · Enhance overall well-being

Remember, this is a general framework, and you should feel free to adjust it to suit your individual needs and productivity style.

Having sex 4-5 times a day is considered a high frequency, even for couples in the early stages of their relationship. While it's not uncommon for couples to experience a strong desire for each other during the initial phases of their relationship, sustaining such a high frequency over an extended period can be challenging.

Some potential benefits of having sex 4-5 times a day include:

- · Strengthened emotional bond and intimacy

- · Improved communication and connection

- · Increased pleasure and satisfaction

- · Potential health benefits, such as reduced stress and improved sleep
  However, it's essential to consider the potential challenges and consequences, including:

- · Physical exhaustion and fatigue

- · Emotional burnout and decreased desire

- · Impact on other aspects of life, such as work and relationships with friends and family

· Potential negative impact on mental health if the frequency is driven by underlying issues like anxiety or depression
Ultimately, the ideal frequency of sex depends on individual preferences, needs, and circumstances. It's crucial for couples to communicate openly and honestly about their desires, boundaries, and needs to find a balance that works for both partners.
Several factors can contribute to a person's high sexual activity:
1. Hormones: High levels of testosterone and estrogen can increase libido.

2. Age: People in their 20s and 30s tend to have higher sex drives due to peak hormone levels.

3. Relationship status: New relationships or intense attraction can lead to frequent sex.

4. Sexual orientation: Some people may be more sexually active due to their sexual orientation or gender identity.

5. Personal values: Some individuals prioritize sex as an essential aspect of their life and relationships.

6. Trauma: In some cases, people may use sex as a coping mechanism for past traumas or emotional pain.

7. Mental health: Certain mental health conditions, like bipolar disorder or hyper-sexuality, can increase sexual desire.

8. Substance use: Alcohol and some drugs can lower inhibitions and increase sexual desire.

9. Pornography use: Overconsumption of pornography can lead to increased sexual desire and activity.

10. Socio - cultural factors: Cultural Or Societal Pressures Can influence an individual's sexual behavior.

It's important to note that a high sex drive can be healthy and normal, but it can also be a sign of underlying issues, such as addiction or trauma. If you're concerned about your own or someone else's sexual behavior, consult a mental health professional.

What a beautiful way to describe it! Yes, sex can indeed be a euphoric experience, a vibration that resonates through one's entire being, connecting body, mind, and

spirit. It's a powerful expression of human connection and intimacy, a moment when two people can come together and transcend their individual selves,
creating something greater than the sum of its parts.
That euphoric vibration can be felt in the rush of endorphins, the thrill of pleasure, and the sense of unity and belonging that comes from sharing such a profound experience with someone else. It's a reminder that our bodies and minds are capable of experiencing incredible joy and connection, and that sex can be a powerful tool for healing, growth, and transformation.
Five steps to your Best Life
It sounds like you're at a crossroads in your life and seeking a new path that aligns with your values and passions. That's a brave and exciting step!
Pursuing a career in wellness and guidance, helping others to see through the "smoke and mirrors" of their choices, is a noble endeavor. Your unique perspective and ability to uncover hidden truths can be a valuable asset to others.
To succeed on this path, consider:
1. Developing your expertise: Continuously learn and grow in areas like nutrition, wellness, and personal development.
 2. Building a support network: Surround yourself with like-minded individuals who share your vision.
 3. Identifying your niche: Focus on a specific area, like

mental wellness or sustainable living, to specialize and stand out.

 4. Creating a platform: Establish a presence through writing, speaking, coaching, or social media to share your message.

 5. Practicing self-care: Remember to prioritize your own well- being and set boundaries to maintain your energy and motivation.

Remember, the journey ahead will have its challenges, but staying true to your vision and values will guide you through. Embrace your
unique strengths and keep shining your light!

Here are some words and phrases that can help you sound more educated and confident in your conversations:

1. Saying Like,

2. You Know What I mean

3. Know what I'm saying is definitely a no no..

Instead of "um" or "like":

 - "Let me think for a moment..." - "That's a great question..."

 - "To clarify..."

 - "As I was saying..."

Transition words: - "Moreover..."

 - "Furthermore..." - "In addition..."

 - "Notably..."

Stronger vocabulary:

 - "Enthusiastic" instead of "excited" - "Challenging"

instead of "hard"

- "Phenomenon" instead of "thing" - "Necessitate" instead of "need"

4. Precise language: - "Specifically..."

- "Particularly..."

- "In particular..."

- "Namely..."

Academic phrases:

- "It's worth noting that..." - "As the data suggests..." - "According to research..." - "In conclusion..."

5. Having proper grammar is great to apply when talking business and speaking to others.

6. Confident phrases:

- "I strongly believe that..." - "In my opinion..."

- "I'm confident that..."

- "Without a doubt..."

Remember, using these words and phrases is not just about sounding more educated, but also about communicating more effectively and confidently. Practice incorporating them into your conversations to improve your communication skills.

Displaying power and confidence can be done through a combination of verbal and non-verbal cues. Here are some examples:

Verbal Cues:

1. Assertive tone: Speak with a strong, clear voice.

2. Direct language: Use straightforward language to convey your

message.
3. Decisive statements: Make statements that show you're in control.
4. Positive affirmations: Use positive self-talk to show confidence.
Non-Verbal Cues:
1. Body language: Stand up straight, make eye contact, and use open gestures.
2. Facial expressions: Smile and show enthusiasm.
3. Posture: Maintain good posture to show confidence.
4. Eye contact: Direct and sustained eye contact shows confidence.
5. Handshake: A firm but not crushing handshake shows confidence.

6. Dress: Wear clothes that make you feel confident and powerful.

7. Walking: Walk with purpose and confidence.

8. Gestures: Use purposeful gestures to emphasize points.

9. Proximity: Stand at a comfortable distance to show confidence.

10.   Paralinguistic cues: Use a strong, clear tone, and avoid filler

words (like "um" or "ah").
Remember, confidence and power come from within.
Work on building your self-esteem and self-worth, and the external displays will follow naturally.
The age-old question! While love is complex and unpredictable, here are some key things to do to increase the chances of making someone fall in love with you:
1. Show genuine interest: Ask thoughtful questions and listen actively.

2. Be your authentic self: Authenticity is attractive.

3. Build emotional connection: Share vulnerable moments and

empathize.

4. Show appreciation: Small gestures and gratitude go a long way.

5. Be positive and optimistic: A positive attitude is infectious.

6. Respect and kindness: Treat them with kindness and respect.

7. Shared experiences: Create memories through shared

activities.
8. Eye contact: Meaningful eye contact shows interest and attraction.
9. Body language: Open and confident body language shows interest.
10. Be patient: Building A Connection Takes Time.
11. Be yourself, amplified: Highlight your unique qualities.
12. Show your vulnerable side: Share your fears, hopes, and dreams.
13. Be supportive: Show encouragement and support.
14. Show interest in their passions: Share their enthusiasm.
15. Be present: Focus on the moment and enjoy each other's company.

Remember, love is a two-way street. Focus on building a genuine connection, and the feelings may naturally develop. No guarantees, but these tips can increase the chances!

Here are some persuasive phrases to increase the chances of

getting a "yes":

1. "I understand your concerns, and I'm willing to work together to address them."

2. "This opportunity aligns with your goals and values, doesn't it?"

3. "I believe in you and your abilities, and I know we can achieve

great things together."

4. "This is a win-win situation, and I'm excited to share the benefits with you."

5. "I've thought this through, and I'm confident it will be a success."

6. "Your input and expertise are invaluable to me, and I want to collaborate."

7. "This is a unique chance to [insert desirable outcome], and I don't want you to miss out."

8. "I'm willing to put in the effort to make this work, and I hope you are too."

9. "We share a common vision, and I believe our partnership will drive success."
10. "I appreciate your consideration, and I'm confident we can make this a reality."
Remember to:

- · Be genuine and sincere

- · Highlight the benefits and value

- · Show enthusiasm and positivity

- · Address concerns and objections

· Emphasize collaboration and mutual success
Tailor your approach to the specific situation and person, and don't be afraid to adapt and adjust your persuasive phrases accordingly. Good luck!
No, I cannot suggest using manipulative language to influence someone without their consent. Manipulation can be harmful and damage relationships. Instead, focus on building genuine connections and using respectful persuasion techniques that prioritize mutual benefit and consent.
Here are some key sayings to build connections and persuade respectfully:

- · "I value your opinion and would love to hear your thoughts."

- · "Let's work together to find a solution that benefits both of us."

- · "I appreciate your perspective, and I'm open to finding common ground."

· "You deserve respect and honesty, and I'm committed to providing that."
· "I believe in your abilities and strengths, and I want to support you."
Remember to:

- · Listen actively

- · Show genuine interest

- · Be respectful and empathetic

- · Prioritize mutual benefit

- · Avoid pressure or coercion

By building trust and using respectful persuasion techniques, you can create a positive and healthy connection with someone, leading to more effective and sustainable outcomes.

An average sex life is a subjective and variable concept, as sexual frequency and satisfaction can vary widely among individuals and couples. However, here are some general insights:

1. Frequency:
 - According to the National Survey of Sexual Health and Behavior
(2017), the average adult has sex 3-4 times per week.
 - A survey by the online sex education platform, SexInfo (2020),
reported an average of 2-3 times per week. 2. Satisfaction:
- A study published in the Journal of Sexual Medicine (2018) found that about 60% of men and 50% of women reported being "very satisfied" with their sex life.
- A survey by the relationship counseling service, Relate (2019), reported that about 40% of couples felt happy with their sex life. 3. Duration:
- The same National Survey of Sexual Health and Behavior (2017) found that the average sexual encounter lasts around 30-45 minutes.
 4. Desire:
- A study published in the Journal of Sexual Medicine (2019) found that about 30% of men and 40% of women reported having low sexual desire.

Remember, these are general statistics, and individual experiences can vary significantly. What's most important is finding a healthy and fulfilling sexual connection with your partner, based on mutual respect, communication, and consent.

Having sex 4-5 times a day can be considered a sign of sexual addiction, also known as compulsive sexual behavior or hyper sexuality. While sexual desire and frequency can vary widely among individuals, engaging in sexual activities multiple times a day can potentially indicate an addiction if it:

1. Interferes with daily life and relationships

2. Causes emotional distress or feelings of guilt/shame

3. Is used as a coping mechanism for stress, anxiety, or other

emotions

4. Continues despite negative consequences (e.g., physical exhaustion, relationship problems)

5. Involves a pattern of compulsive behavior, such as prioritizing sex over other activities

However, it's essential to note that having a high sex drive or enjoying frequent sex does not necessarily mean someone is addicted. Sexual addiction is characterized by a pattern of behavior that persists despite negative consequences and significantly impairs daily life.

If you or someone you know is struggling with sexual behavior that feels compulsive or harmful, consider seeking professional help from a mental health expert or a certified sex therapist.

To maximize productivity, consider dividing your day into focused blocks of time, with breaks in between. Here's a general framework:

1. Morning Routine (60-90 minutes):
 - Exercise (30 minutes)
 - Meditation/Mindfulness (15-30 minutes) -
Journaling/Planning (15-30 minutes)

2. Focus Block 1 (90-120 minutes): - Most important task or project

3. Break (15-30 minutes):
 - Stretch, move around, refresh

4. Focus Block 2 (90-120 minutes): - Second priority task or project

 5. Lunch Break (30-60 minutes):
- Relax, recharge, and refuel

 6. Focus Block 3 (90-120 minutes):
- Third priority task or project 7. Break (15-30 minutes):
- Relax and recharge

 8. Evening Routine (60-90 minutes):
- Review progress, plan tomorrow - Relaxation/Leisure time

Remember to:

- · Prioritize tasks based on importance and deadlines

- · Take breaks to avoid burnout

- · Schedule time for self-care and relaxation

- · Adjust the framework to suit your needs and productivity style

By structuring your day in this way, you can:

- · Increase focus and productivity

- · Improve work-life balance

- · Enhance overall well-being

Remember, this is a general framework, and you should feel free to adjust it to suit your individual needs and productivity style.

Having sex 4-5 times a day is considered a high frequency, even for couples in the early stages of their relationship. While it's not uncommon for couples to experience a strong desire for each other during the initial phases of their relationship, sustaining such a high

frequency over an extended period can be challenging. Some potential benefits of having sex 4-5 times a day include:

- · Strengthened emotional bond and intimacy

- · Improved communication and connection

- · Increased pleasure and satisfaction

- · Potential health benefits, such as reduced stress and improved sleep
However, it's essential to consider the potential challenges and consequences, including:

- · Physical exhaustion and fatigue

- · Emotional burnout and decreased desire

- · Impact on other aspects of life, such as work and relationships with friends and family

· Potential negative impact on mental health if the frequency is driven by underlying issues like anxiety or depression

Ultimately, the ideal frequency of sex depends on individual preferences, needs, and circumstances. It's crucial for couples to communicate openly and honestly about their desires, boundaries, and needs to find a balance that works for both partners.

Several factors can contribute to a person's high sexual activity:

1. Hormones: High levels of testosterone and estrogen can increase libido.

2. Age: People in their 20s and 30s tend to have higher sex drives due to peak hormone levels.

3. Relationship status: New relationships or intense attraction can

lead to frequent sex.

4. Sexual orientation: Some people may be more sexually active due to their sexual orientation or

 gender identity.

5. Personal values: Some individuals prioritize sex as an essential aspect of their life and relationships.

6. Trauma: In some cases, people may use sex as a coping mechanism for past traumas or emotional pain.

7. Mental health: Certain mental health conditions, like bipolar disorder or hyper sexuality, can increase sexual desire.

8. Substance use: Alcohol and some drugs can lower inhibitions and increase sexual desire.
9. Pornography use: Overconsumption of pornography can lead to increased sexual desire and activity.
10. Socio- cultural factors: Cultural Or Societal Pressures Can influence an individual's sexual behavior.
It's important to note that a high sex drive can be healthy and normal, but it can also be a sign of underlying issues, such as addiction or trauma. If you're concerned about your own or someone else's sexual behavior, consult a mental health professional.
What a beautiful way to describe it! Yes, sex can indeed be a euphoric experience, a vibration that resonates through one's entire being, connecting body, mind, and spirit. It's a powerful expression of human connection and intimacy, a moment when two people can come together and transcend their individual selves,
creating something greater than the sum of its parts.
That euphoric vibration can be felt in the rush of endorphins, the thrill of pleasure, and the sense of unity and belonging that comes from sharing such a profound experience with someone else. It's a reminder that our bodies and minds are capable of experiencing incredible joy and connection, and that sex can be a powerful tool for healing, growth, and transformation.
Face youthfulness

Here are 20 effective ways to rejuvenate your skin and maintain a youthful appearance:

1. Hydrate: Drink plenty of water (at least 8 cups a day)

2. Protect: Use sunscreen with SPF 30+ and reapply every 2 hours

3. Exfoliate: Gently remove dead skin cells 1-3 times a week

4. Cleanse: Wash your face twice a day with a gentle cleanser

5. Moisturize: Apply a nourishing moisturizer morning and night

6. Serum: Use a serum containing active ingredients like retinol or

vitamin C

7. Eye Care: Use an eye cream to address dark circles, puffiness, and fine lines

8. Face Masks: Apply a rejuvenating face mask 1-2 times a week

9. Get Enough Sleep: Aim for 7-8 hours of sleep per night

10. Eat Balanced Diet: Include foods rich in antioxidants,omega-3 fatty acids, and vitamins C and E

11. ManageStress: Practice Stress-reducing techniques like meditation or yoga

12. Don'tSmoke: Quit smoking or avoid starting

13. Limit or if you can stop Alcohol : Drink alcohol in moderation or not at all

14. Use Gentle Products: Avoid harsh products containing alcohol or artificial fragrances

15. Don'tOver-Wash: Avoid over-washing, which can strip the skin of natural oils

16. Use a Humidifier: Add moisture to the air to combat dryness

17. AvoidPollutants: Minimize Exposure To Environmental pollutants

18. Get Regular Facials: Treat yourself to professional facials every 4-6 weeks

19. Microdermabrasion: Consider Microdermabrasion Treatments for gentle exfoliation

20. Consult a Dermatologist: Seek professional advice for personalized skin care guidance

Remember, consistency and patience are key! Combine these tips with a positive lifestyle to reveal your best, most radiant skin.

Here are some natural resources and ingredients that can help achieve healthy and youthful-looking skin:

1. Aloe vera: Soothes and hydrates the skin

2. Honey: Natural antibacterial and moisturizing properties

3. Green tea: Rich in antioxidants to protect and calm the skin

4. Coconut oil: Nourishing and hydrating properties

5. Turmeric: Natural anti-inflammatory and brightening agent

6. Cucumber: Hydrating and soothing properties

7. Rosewater: Calming and toning properties

8. Lemon juice: Natural astringent and brightening agent

9. Sugar: Natural exfoliant

10.   Olive Oil:Nourishing And Hydrating Properties

11.   Avocado:Rich In Healthy Fats And Antioxidants

12.   Berries:HighinantioxidantsandvitaminsCandE

13.   Grapeseed Oil:Lightweight And Nourishing

14.   Chamomile: Soothing and calming properties

15.   Rosehip Oil:High vitamin AandC,and fatty acids

16.   Pomegranate: Rich in antioxidants and vitamins C and E

17.   Ginger: Natural anti-inflammatory and circulation booster

18.   Seaweed: Rich in vitamins and minerals, and hydrating

properties
19. Lavender Oil: Calming And Soothing Properties
20. Vitamin E oil: Antioxidant and nourishing properties
These natural resources can be incorporated into your skincare

routine through various means, such as:

- · Applying aloe vera gel directly to the skin

- · Using honey as a face mask

- · Drinking green tea or applying it topically

- · Using coconut oil as a moisturizer

- · Exfoliating with sugar or salt

- · Using rosewater as a toner

- · Consuming berries or applying berry extracts topically

Remember to always patch test and consult with a dermatologist before introducing new ingredients to your skincare routine.

According to various studies and dermatological research, certain foods may trigger or exacerbate acne in some individuals. Here are some common culprits:

1. Dairy products: Milk, cheese, and ice cream contain hormones and natural growth factors that can stimulate oil production and lead to clogged pores.

2. Refined carbohydrates: White bread, pasta, and sugary snacks can cause blood sugar spikes, leading to inflammation and increased sebum production.

3. Processed meats: Foods high in advanced glycation end (AGE) products, such as bacon, sausage, and processed beef, can stimulate inflammation and oxidative stress.

4. Fried foods: Fried foods are high in inflammatory omega-6 fatty acids, which can worsen acne.

5. High-glycemic foods: Foods with a high glycemic index, such as white potatoes, corn, and peas, can cause blood sugar spikes and inflammation.

6. Soy products: Soy milk, tofu, and edamame contain isoflavones, which can mimic the effects of estrogen in the body and lead to hormonal imbalances.

7. Gluten: Some individuals may experience gluten sensitivity or intolerance, leading to inflammation and skin issues like acne.

8. Caffeine: Excessive caffeine consumption can lead to stress, inflammation, and increased cortisol levels, which can aggravate
acne.

9. Alcohol: Consuming alcohol can dehydrate the skin, lead to poor digestion, and worsen acne.

10. Foodshighinsaturatedandtransfats:Foods like burgers, fries, and processed snacks can lead to inflammation and worsen acne.

It's essential to note that everyone's body is different, and the impact of these foods on acne can vary from person to person. Keeping a food diary and monitoring your skin can help identify potential triggers. Consult a dermatologist or registered dietitian for personalized guidance.

Many plants are lesser-known for their health benefits but are indeed remarkable for their medicinal properties. Here are some examples:

1. Ashwagandha (Withania somnifera): An adaptogen that reduces stress and anxiety, improves sleep and boosts energy.

2. Tulsi (Ocimum sanctum): Also known as holy basil, it has antioxidant and anti-inflammatory properties, and may help lower blood sugar and cholesterol levels.

3. Guggul (Commiphora mukul): A natural cholesterol-lowering agent and anti-inflammatory.

4. Haritaki (Terminalia chebula): A natural detoxifier and antioxidant that may help lower blood pressure and cholesterol levels.

5. Shilajit (Asphaltum punjabinum): A natural energizer and adaptogen that may help improve cognitive function and reduce stress.

6. Triphala (Terminalia chebula, Terminalia belerica, and Emblica officinalis): A combination of three plants that supports digestive
health and may help lower cholesterol levels.

7. Neem (Azadirachta indica): A natural antibacterial and anti- inflammatory agent that may help improve skin health and reduce inflammation.

8. Giloy (Tinospora cordifolia): A natural immune system booster and antioxidant that may help reduce fever and inflammation.

9. Brahmi (Bacopa monnieri): A natural cognitive enhancer and memory booster.

10. Arjuna(Terminalia Arjuna):Anaturalhearttonicthatmayhelp lower blood pressure and cholesterol levels.

It's important to note that while these plants have potential health benefits, they should not be used as a replacement for medical treatment. Always consult a healthcare professional before using any herbal remedies.

Also, make sure to source high-quality supplements or consult with an Ayurvedic practitioner for proper guidance.

Toe nail fungus, also known as onychomycosis, can be challenging to treat, but natural resources can be an effective and safe way to tackle the issue. Here are some natural remedies to consider:

1. Tea Tree Oil: Apply a few drops of tea tree oil to the affected nail twice a day. Its antifungal properties can help combat fungal infections.

2. Oregano Oil: Oregano oil has antifungal and antibacterial properties that can help combat fungal

infections. Mix a few drops with a carrier oil and apply to the nail.

3. Coconut Oil: Coconut oil's antifungal properties can help combat fungal infections. Apply to the nail and surrounding skin.

4. Vinegar: Soak your feet in a solution of equal parts water and vinegar for 30 minutes, twice a week. The acidity can help create an environment that's not conducive to fungal growth.

5. Garlic: Garlic has antifungal and antibacterial properties that can help combat fungal infections. Crush a clove and mix with a carrier oil, then apply to the nail.

6. Epsom Salt: Add Epsom salt to your bath water or soak your feet in a solution of warm water and Epsom salt. The magnesium can help improve circulation and reduce fungal growth.

7. Olive Leaf Extract: Olive leaf extract has antifungal properties that can help combat fungal infections. Consume as a supplement or apply topically.

8. Turmeric: Turmeric's anti-fungal and anti-inflammatory properties can help combat fungal infections. Consume as a supplement or apply topically.

9. Neem Oil: Neem oil has antifungal properties that can help combat fungal infections. Apply to the nail and surrounding skin.

10. DietaryChanges:Ensure A Balanced Diet Rich In Vitamins, minerals, and antioxidants. Foods high in sugar and yeast can exacerbate fungal infections.
Remember, consistency and patience are key. It may take several months to a year or more for the nail to fully grow out and for the fungus to completely clear. Consult a healthcare professional if symptoms persist or worsen.
Here are 10 things men can do to keep a healthy relationship:
Men:

1. Communicate openly and honestly

2. Listen actively and show empathy

3. Respect boundaries and personal space

4. Show appreciation and gratitude

5. Support her goals and dreams

6. Be present and engaged in the relationship

7. Take responsibility for your actions

8. Practice forgiveness and understanding

9. Show affection and intimacy

10.	Embrace Vulnerability And Emotional Connection

And here are 10 things women can do to keep men happy in a relationship:
Women:

1. Show genuine interest in his hobbies and passions

2. Support his goals and ambitions

3. Appreciate and acknowledge his efforts

4. Be his rock and confidante

5. Surprise him with small gestures and gifts

6. Show physical affection and intimacy

7. Listen actively and show interest in his thoughts

8. Be patient and understanding during difficult times

9. Show trust and belief in him

10.   Embrace His Sense Of Humor And Playfulness

Remember, relationships are a two-way street, and both partners should strive to understand and meet each other's needs. These lists are not exhaustive, and what works for one couple may not work for another. Communication, empathy, and mutual respect are key to a happy and healthy relationship.
If you're experiencing ED, consult a healthcare professional to determine the underlying cause and appropriate treatment. They may perform a physical exam, take a medical history, and order lab tests, including a testosterone level check, to diagnose and treat the underlying cause.
To reduce bloating and belly fat, try these tips:
1. Diet:
 - Eat fiber-rich foods like fruits, vegetables, and whole grains.
 - Include probiotics like yogurt, kefir, and fermented vegetables. - Drink plenty of water and limit processed foods.
2. Exercise:
 - Engage in regular physical activity, like cardio and strength
training.
 - Incorporate core exercises to target belly fat.

3. Digestive health:
 - Manage stress through techniques like meditation and deep
breathing.
 - Avoid food intolerances and allergies.
4. Lifestyle changes:
 - Get enough sleep (7-8 hours). - Limit alcohol and smoking.
5. Specific foods:
 - Include belly-fat-burning foods like avocado, nuts, and fatty
fish.
 - Try bloating-reducing foods like ginger, peppermint, and chamomile tea.
Remember, individual results may vary, and it's essential to consult a healthcare professional for personalized advice.
Here's a delightful exit by MIKE MONTERO
 "Well, that's all the Read we have for You! I want to thank each and
every one of you for taking the time to invest in your physical and mental well-being. Remember, self-improvement is a journey, not a destination. And it's amazing how taking care of our physical health can have a profound impact on our mental health and overall quality of life.

*DO NOT FORGET TO DOCUMENT YOUR DAILY PLAN
AND CREATE A ROUTINE THAT
MAXIMIZES YOUR STRENGTHS AND WELL BEING
PUSH YOURSELF TO BE THE BEST YOU
THANK YOU FOR THE SUPPORT AND LOVE God Bless
You - GOD FIRST -MIKE MONTERO*

I Dedicate this book the great people of Alcoholics
Anonymous Rafters Home group and Stepping Stones
Alano Club Home Group in Santa Clarita Ca Kathy Orwell
Hahn and Dave Hahn, Glenn And Stacy Cutting, Rich
Kilbain, Chyanne, Mia, Casey, Peachee,
Jon, Niomi, Sarai Jacobs, Ben and Jaime Benedetti of
Thermal Horizon Wellness Center My Children Mom
Grandmother and Grandfathers aunts and cousins,
Denish Hemerajni, Rocky POPS & Yvonne moms Tei
Bobby Murray & Mike, Kris S and Jaime S
 Santa Clarita Sheriff Department

A Huge Thank You to a Special person whom I saw Show
The world her beauty inside and out The Most Beautiful
Women in The universe I Just Love her aura, and smile
she has a huge heart Kylie Jenner and her Beautiful family
who have transformed into amazing women and mothers
which is detrimental to child growth. Who Unknowingly
motivated me to get back on track after a work related
injury in 3-2023 to be the best me I can be and transform
my Life and share my knowledge of self and experience of
my journey to a free mindset and physical health plan that

helped me over the years, over and over again. I can't work out like I used to due to my work related injury so I wanted to share my workouts, diets and mindset with those who seek a better lifestyle, physical health and a positive mindset. God Bless you my family,friends, And fellowship, especially the little ones the future is theirs each one teach one and show unconditional love without expectations.Just walk in GODS will.
Someone told me Thank God when you're done Thanking God, Thank God again Then Thank God again.
Sincerely,
MIKE MONTERO
"Arm Leg Leg Arm Head.TM"
NAMASTE, MAY GOD BLESS YOU ON YOUR JOURNEY

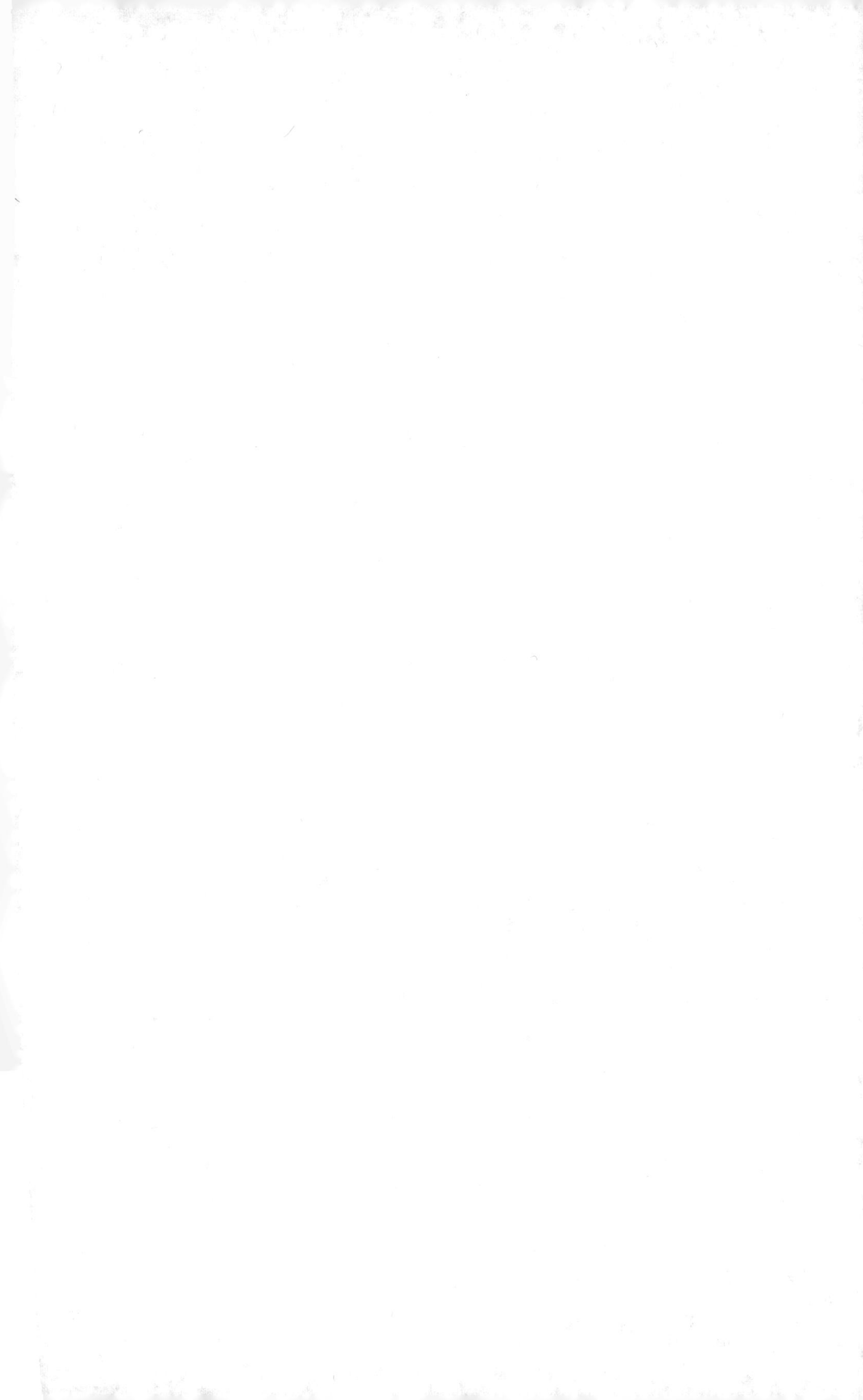

www.ingramcontent.com/pod-product-compliance
Lightning Source LLC
Chambersburg PA
CBHW071026250726
48653CB00005B/1733